The Outer You...
The Inner You

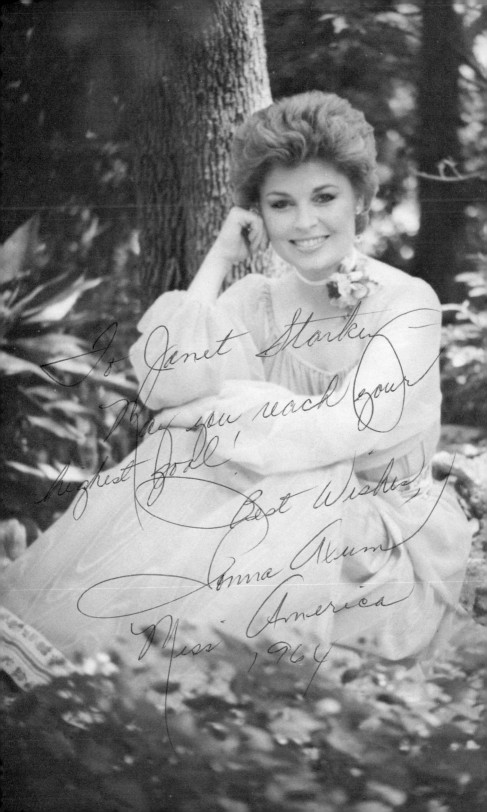

To Janet Starkey
May you reach your
highest goal!
Best Wishes,
Donna Axum
Miss America
1964

The Outer You...
The Inner You

Donna Axum

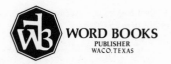

WORD BOOKS
PUBLISHER
WACO, TEXAS

Frontispiece photo: Christianson Leberman House of Portraits

First Printing – March 1978
Second Printing – May 1978

THE OUTER YOU . . . THE INNER YOU
Copyright © 1978 by Word, Incorporated, Waco, Texas 76703.
All rights reserved.
No portion of this book may be
reproduced in any form, except for brief
quotations in reviews, without the
written permission of the
publisher.

Scripture quotations marked TLB
are from *The Living Bible, Paraphrased*
(Wheaton: Tyndale House Publishers, 1971)
and are used by permission

ISBN 0–8499–0055–7
Library of Congress catalog card number: 77–83345
Printed in the United States of America

*To my loved ones and
all those who have touched
my life in a meaningful way*

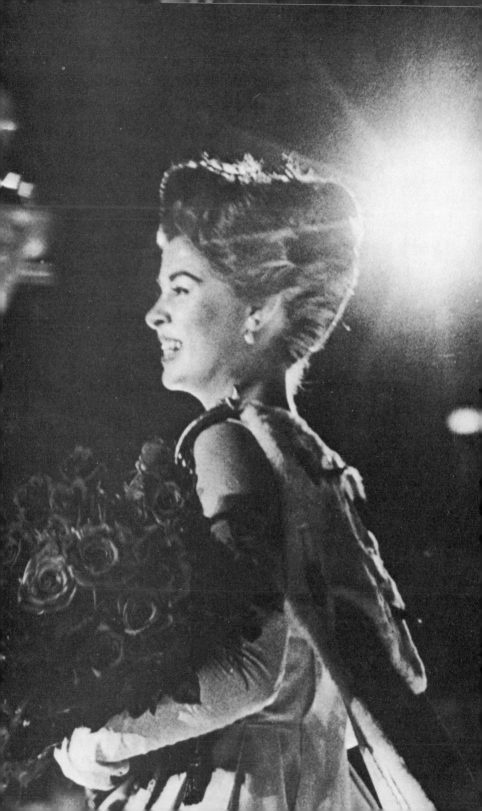

Contents

Introduction

Knowing how to swim is not only fun but can also save you from drowning. And one of the first things that you learn is how to tread water. This enables you to keep your head above water for extended periods of time without moving in any direction.

Have you ever reached a point in your life when you've felt you were at a standstill, confused, not knowing which direction to take—just "treading water"?

Sitting in my office at the University of Texas one day in the spring of 1975, I realized that was what I was doing. As I thought about my life and where I was headed, I knew I was not utilizing all my experiences and talents. It was time, once again, to stop treading water, make some decisions, and start moving again.

I was a 33-year-old divorced working mother and a former Miss America, all wrapped into a single person. I had experienced the heights of glamor and success. I had also known the depression of failure and the helpless despair of innocent involvement in the worst political scandal in recent Texas history.

As I looked at my life, I realized that there was much in my background that could be of unique value to other

9

women. I began to compile a list of the major events and experiences of my life. It looked like this:
- —Participation in 16 pageants leading up to the titles
- —Miss Arkansas and Miss America of 1964
- —Extensive experience in radio and TV, modeling, speaking, and pageant emcee work
- —Bachelor of Arts degree, University of Arkansas
- —Master of Arts degree, University of Arkansas
- —Postgraduate study, University of Texas, Austin
- —College and university teaching and counseling
- —Two marriages and divorces
- —Two children
- —Several catastrophes: 6-point earthquake in Mexico City; hotel fire in Florida; the first "blackout" in New York City
- —Father's death from cancer
- —Two rounds of major surgery
- —Husband's state political scandal: trial; harassment

As I pondered my list, I also remembered a charm and modeling course I had taught some eight years earlier. I thought how different that course would be if I had the opportunity to speak to women today. Coping with problems in my life during the intervening years has given me some new insights into the importance of inner beauty and strength. I know that my life now has a depth that it did not have before. I wanted to share all of my experiences and new insights with other women with the hope that they could relate it to their lives and grow.

From this thinking, I began to develop the concept of the Outer You and the Inner You, a personal development course that I taught in Austin. The Inner You deals with the idea that the real beauty of a woman lies inside her heart and mind; the Outer You is based on the idea that there are practical tools through which every woman can capture the unique, individual outer beauty that is rightfully hers. I have tried to present here principles of diet, exercise, make-up, hair care, wardrobe, and visual poise that can help women to accomplish God's purpose for their lives and to cope with the challenges of ever-expanding roles in society.

As the School of Communication Job Placement Director at the University of Texas, Austin, I was distressed to talk to recent graduates with degrees in hand who had little thought for tomorrow. Through counseling I also saw the frustration of the middle-aged woman wishing for a degree or meaningful career but thinking that perhaps it was too late. For these women and all others between the two extremes the Christian message is: it's never too late to commit yourself to a fresh start.

The Outer You—The Inner You provides practical guidelines for self-renewal and improvement. Look at them and apply them as they fit you. I am not selling any one approach or way of thinking. Neither am I suggesting that every woman should seek a career or that everyone should look like a model. Rather, I believe that every woman reaches crucial times when she must critically evaluate her life, make decisions, set goals, and move forward.

It is my hope that this book will help women to better accept themselves, to identify and develop talents, and to turn their energies and abilities outward—to achieve high self-esteem. Some women cope better than others. Many don't utilize their talents to reach their fullest potential. They are caught in ruts of routine from which they lack the knowledge or the courage to extricate themselves. Still others are insecure and overly concerned about their looks and general impression. Women who cannot forget themselves and focus on others have difficulty in giving and loving. Their world is small because it is completely dominated by "I" instead of "you."

If any of the things I have just mentioned strike a familiar note, take this book and proceed to build yourself as an individual. You *can* develop self-assurance and esteem, but it must begin with an honest evaluation and a positive commitment. Take a close look at yourself. Identify what you can contribute to those around you—your friends, family, business associates, church. Everyone has assets. You can learn to use yours: just try! You can move out of the darkness into the sunlight and make your life more meaningful, fulfilling, and rewarding. Be a "mover"—only you can make it happen!

There's one other thing I'd like to share, and it's very important. The Bible has been a motivating force in my life (I trust it will be in yours too), so you will find a number of Bible quotations in this book. This one just happens to be one of my favorites and one that has helped me immeasurably through the years: "I can do all things through Christ which strengtheneth me" (Phil. 4:13).

The Outer You

☙ 1 ❧

Visual Poise—The Non-Verbal You

You never get a second chance to make a good first impression! The old adage tells us never to judge a book by its cover, yet we still find ourselves attracted to an eye-catching book jacket or repelled by a visually disturbing one. This is not to say that some of the best reading material can't be found in the pages of a drab-looking book, but simply to recognize the power of what pleases the eye. Right or wrong, first impressions are very important, and people do assume that the outer you that they see is a fairly good indication of the qualities and characteristics the inner you possesses.

The first impression we make on others is usually communicated non-verbally through our carriage, the way we walk and sit, our gestures and mannerisms, as well as our general grooming. It is also conveyed in the way we enter a room, the way we stand, the way we hold our head, the way we hold our shoulders. These things say something very important about how we feel about ourselves. It is a tremendous compliment for someone to say about another woman, "She has such beautiful carriage." Here's a person who feels good about herself, he is saying—someone who is sure of herself, knows who she is and where she's going. In contrast, the shy, insecure person is very often someone who doesn't

hold her head up, who has difficulty looking people in the
eye and who walks around as though she is carrying the
whole world on her shoulders.

This analysis does not always prove correct, of course.
But what I am saying is this: our bodies talk, and the world
has become accustomed to reading that language. Wouldn't
we rather have someone read self-confidence and a healthy
self-esteem in the way we stand, walk and sit, than careless-
ness, depression, and a lack of self-assurance? We are attracted to the individual who radiates a happy sense of
well-being, confidence and positive attitude through good
posture, body handling, and facial expressions.

Grace of body and movement is something one achieves
by recognition, first of all, that it is important and worth
understanding. Once a woman realizes that her body tells
others a lot about herself, she has taken a giant step. She
will not only be able to improve her image, but also her
general sense of well-being and health. The rewards will be
great in several different areas.

It's never too late to learn how to stand, walk, and sit
correctly. Not only are you going to look better to others
and yourself, but you are going to feel better psychologically and physically. Everyone really wants to be well
received by others. Acceptance by others generates self-
acceptance and goes a long way toward building self-confidence and self-esteem. I like this little maxim learned from
a friend who was working on self-improvement while trying
not to be overly self-indulgent in the process: "I have to
live with myself and so, I want to be fit for myself to know."

She was being very wise. You do yourself *and others* a
favor when you think well of yourself. That's a biblical concept; Jesus himself offered the eleventh commandment,
Thou shalt love the Lord thy God and thy neighbor *as thy-
self*. As we talk more about the outer you and the inner you,
we shall be thinking in terms of this kind of *proper* self-love
and ways to help bring it about. (Notice my emphasis on
proper.)

Let's begin with the way we project ourselves to others—
the outer you. Allan Fromme, in his book *The Ability to
Love*, states that "the more kindly we judge ourselves, the

more kindly we are in judging others. The more we accept ourselves, with all our defects and shortcomings, the more acceptance we can offer to those we love. Anyone unhappy with himself is easily sullen and irritable with others."

Are you happy with yourself? Are you happy with the way you walk? The way you sit? What about your carriage? If not, then (let's begin with the basics) make the first major decision that you *want* to improve and will dedicate yourself to that end.

The first thing to learn in developing good carriage is correct body alignment.

Slumping and generally poor posture give the impression of weakness—that you're a loser.

Good posture indicates strength—a winner.

CORRECT BODY ALIGNMENT

If the organs in your body are functioning correctly, you are going to feel good. Holding our bodies in correct alignment when we stand and when we sit is a beautiful art we need to master. When we are slumped over or stooped, we are mashing down on the stomach and other internal organs. We are causing ourselves all kinds of difficulty in breathing, for instance; because of being squeezed, our lungs and our diaphragm do not work at top efficiency. Doesn't it make good sense to recognize that when we do stand up straight and hold our body correctly, everything within it can function and work together as God designed it?

Are you wondering how you can establish what is *your* body's correct alignment? (For those of you entering beauty pageants this is the first place to start in your presentation on stage and off.) Here is how I do it.

Step I—Good Carriage

I stand with my back against the wall and touch my head, my shoulders (pushing them all the way back), and my backbone to it as nearly as possible. (This will be difficult if you are swayback.) Then I touch my buttocks and my heels against the wall. This is a very rigid stance, but necessary for determining your correct body alignment.

Next, walk away from the wall and then slightly relax. Do this by letting your shoulders relax—not letting them slump forward, but easing them to the point where you don't look (or feel) like a wooden soldier. Now your body will be in correct alignment, and you should feel comfortable. If I were there I should be able to draw an imaginary straight line down the side of your body through your ears, your shoulders, your hips, your knees and ankles. Have someone check you.

Perhaps at this point you are protesting that this is unreal, there aren't any people who could walk around like that. Oh yes, there are! And these are people who do not develop back or muscle problems. Their backs and their muscles become strong over a period of years. The more you protest, the stronger would be my suspicion that you in particular need to work at developing good body alignment.

If you are not accustomed to standing up straight, your back muscles will tire easily at first; develop them through practice and exercise. This, first of all, is the key to good carriage. The minute you stand straight and sit up straight your whole body will respond, and in time you will not only see but feel the difference. There is an unexpected psychological benefit from this—you will automatically feel stronger about yourself.

Since body alignment is such an important factor in revealing our personality traits to others, we need to be aware that through it we are giving out visual clues about ourselves all the time. The world of public speaking calls this "platform manner." The way a speaker sits on stage and approaches a podium is a key factor in determining how an audience will accept her and respond—even before she opens her mouth to speak. A speaker can set the tone for acceptance or rejection by her knowledge and skill in movement and carriage. This is frequently referred to as poise; my definition of poise is a feeling of confidence in who you are, what you are, where you are going, and your complete control of the situation. We gravitate toward people who reflect self-confidence and poise. The poised individual radiates that certain magic quality which seems to say, "I've got it all together."

A number of women in my development courses have told me they were amazed to realize that standing up straight helps eliminate some of their problems with a bulging stomach and a roll around the midriff. Of course that extra flesh has to go somewhere, and if you are going to slouch you are going to mash it down between your trunk and your torso. But when you stand up straight, you lengthen the space between your torso and your hips, and you straighten out that skin and stretch it up. By pulling in that tummy and getting your body in correct alignment, you can make yourself look five to ten pounds lighter immediately without losing one pound.

I work with young women who are entering beauty pageants and we concentrate very hard in this area. Imagine that you are a marionette and that there is a string holding up your head—not to the point where it is pulling your nose up into the air (because that gives the impression of being haughty) but to the point where you feel almost regal. I would describe it as an uplifted feeling. Then imagine that this string goes right down and is attached to the sternum (the breastbone). If you keep that up and your head up, you will be raising the torso also. This will give you a beautiful bustline and also lengthen your midriff area and get rid of that midriff bulge. Then if you move your head back just slightly on your backbone, you will look truly queenly and regal in a very natural way. Another secret for competition, especially in the swimsuit category: slightly expand and lift the rib cage, as if inhaling. This will lift the bustline area and lengthen and flatten midriff and abdomen area even more.

God intended for us women to look graceful and beautiful. I have found that when I cooperate with the One who designed me in the first place I don't tire as easily; with everything in correct alignment my backbone easily supports the weight of my body. Not only do we harm our muscles when we habitually slouch—whether standing, walking, or sitting—but we constantly increase our chances for body fatigue.

Even women who have a tendency to be swayback—and many do—can help themselves a great deal by following this tip. Practice rotating your pelvic bone forward and tucking under your bottom (the buttocks). Tuck it under, even while standing or walking, as if you were going to sit down in a chair. This will help straighten the spine and pull your body into correct alignment. It should also pull in your protruding midriff area. Needless to say, having the buttocks pulled under instead of sticking out also produces a more ladylike appearance.

Step II—A Beautiful Walk

Few things are more important to the outer you than a beautiful walk and a graceful carriage. Lord Byron painted a striking word portrait: "She walks in beauty, like the night/Of cloudless climes and starry skies." On the other hand, I've witnessed some ladies who looked as if they were following behind a plow in the north forty!

Learning how to walk beautifully is something you can develop. We learn to walk as children, and along the way, many of us develop some bad habits in walking. You may have to unlearn some of these bad habits, but it can be done.

The way a person walks is dictated in part by the length of the legs, since that determines the length of the step, or *stride*. The key to developing a beautiful walk, in my opinion, is the stride. When I work with women, I watch them walk and analyze their stride. Too short a stride is reflected by fast, restricted movements. Too long a stride gives a more masculine, hurried look. Observe for yourself in a long mirror how you walk. When I was preparing for all the various beauty pageants that I entered over the years, some sixteen in all, I am sure I wore out several rugs in walking back and forth down the hall toward the full-length mirror that hung there. I was checking my body alignment and my stride among other things.

A second important factor is *gait*, the rhythm of the steps you take. Whether you are long-legged, short, or in-between, analyze your stride and gait. If possible, get someone in your family to help you in this determination. If you have short legs, perhaps you need to work at lengthening your stride; they may propel you along as if you are always in a hurry. If your legs are long, take proportionate steps accordingly, being careful not to make them overly long or masculine—don't gallop. It also helps to walk as if you know where you are going rather than just to amble along.

A beautiful walk is good posture in pleasing motion. As the poem suggests, "The longest journey starts with a single step," so that's where we will begin.

Step III—The Feet

Let's look at our feet. Do you step correctly? When you walk, your feet should move in parallel motion, pointed straight ahead and only a few inches apart. Center your weight just in front of the ankle and let the heel come down first. Rotate your weight on the outer side of your foot, and then onto your toes, using them to push forward for the next step. As your foot follows through, rotate it to the inside and break your ankle inward. (Breaking your ankle means turning it in, not keeping it rigid.) This allows for the graceful movement of the hips.

What is incorrect stepping and walking? Have you ever seen someone who clump, clump, clumps along? She is putting her whole foot down at once, resulting in that flat-footed, clump, clump, clump. Or she may put the ball of her foot down first and then the heel—I refer to this as the ballerina walk. Or she may noisily drag her feet along.

At the racetrack, comments are frequently made on the beautiful gait of a thoroughbred horse. A woman can develop that same sort of gait. Compare that to the image of an old mare clumping down the street, with every step an excruciating effort.

Step IV—The Knees

One of the keys to a graceful, floating, feminine walk is the action of the knees. Keep your knees slightly flexed. Picture a football player receiving the ball on a kickoff; he doesn't stand there rigid with his arms outstretched, instead his body recoils as he catches it, his knees absorbing the shock. In the same way, think of your knees as springs in your body helping promote the graceful, flowing look that you are seeking to develop. When you take a step, rather than holding your knees straight and rigid, keep them flexible enough to absorb the shock of each step so you won't bounce from the waist up.

Your walking will reflect the fact that your body is in proper alignment. Your head will not be sticking forward, nor will you swing or wriggle your hips in an exaggerated fashion; rather, there will be a graceful and natural side to side movement. With a proper understanding of what it takes, you will find it easier than you think to achieve the graceful feminine image.

Step V—The Hands and Arms

When you are walking, keep in mind that a curved line is far more flattering to a woman than a straight rigid line. Let your hands fall in a loose, natural curve with the fingers relaxed. Your shoulders should be sufficiently relaxed to enable your arms to swing easily, elbows at the side. It is always more flattering to present your hands from a side view. Hold your hands so that the thumb and index fingers are swinging forward rather than the flat part of your hand. Keep your upper arms rather close to your body, and remember that the swinging of your arms should be in correct *opposition* to your steps. Now put all these parts together, and practice, practice, practice.

As you walk, keep your neck up, out of your shoulders. In this way, your chin will be parallel to the floor. This also helps eliminate double chins. Make the image you are projecting the vehicle for your happiness. With some concentrated effort at first, you will soon find that you are doing these things effortlessly and reaping tremendous rewards in terms of both physical and emotional well-being.

Step VI—The Way You Sit

How you approach a chair, sit in it, and get up out of it tells a lot about you! Here are some tips that will make you look better and feel more comfortable. If you have a choice when you walk into a room of a number of different types of chairs (couches, footstools . . .), be good to yourself! Be selfish if need be, particularly if you have ahead of you a long evening or a long session of sitting. Locate a chair that you will fit into comfortably. This is really very important. If you are a short individual, for instance, you shouldn't select a deep sofa or deep chair because, once you get settled into it, you are going to have some difficulty in maneuvering your legs to get up again. Select something that will be comfortable and that will allow for graceful sitting and good posture.

Once you have selected the seat, approach the chair without looking down! No, you don't need to turn around and look behind you to make sure the chair is still there. Don't even look down. Approach the chair, then turn and find the chair with the back of your calf. Then simply lower yourself vertically on the edge of the chair, keeping your torso in good alignment, never once sticking out your bottom! Go straight down, ever so gracefully, avoiding any kind of movement that calls attention to your posterior. As you go down, place one foot slightly behind the other. The next natural movement is to use your hands to lift your body slightly as you ease yourself back into the chair.

We've all seen women drop into a chair, hips first—a most ungraceful movement, and one that widens the hips every time they plop down in that manner. Did you know that when you sit down properly you are giving yourself an exercise that helps firm and tighten the muscles of both your thighs and buttocks? Tuck those hips under, tighten up those muscles, and you'll be doing yourself a favor in more ways than one!

Now, how are you going to sit? A woman sitting properly is a lovely sight to behold! By contrast, what is more distasteful than to see a woman sprawled out? Your body is certainly not communicating "lady."

First of all, you're going to sit straight—no, not ramrod straight, but comfortably erect. Remember good body alignment, and don't let everything mash together.

What are you going to do with your hands, your legs, and your feet? There are a number of variations. The most graceful look, and my own favorite position, is the S curve. (It helps always to remember that anything curved is far more flattering to a woman than straight up and down lines.) The

S curve will give that nice, attractive flowing line to the body. In this S curve position, curl the big toe of one foot behind the ankle of the other as you slant your legs either to the left or right. The important thing is that the leg that is out in front has the instep of that foot angled or parallel to the floor. Now place your hands together comfortably on the top of your thigh.

A physical fitness expert recommends this next variation. Simply put one foot slightly in front of the other with both feet resting squarely on the floor a few inches apart, with the weight slightly on the outer edges. The important feature about any kind of leg position is that you always keep your knees together.

The most unladylike way to sit (as so many overweight women do) is to stick your legs out in front and cross your ankles. Please, no! Pull your legs under you and keep your knees together.

Never cross your legs when being photographed or when sitting on stage before an audience.

For those who feel they must cross their legs, there is one better way of doing so than any other. The *wrong* way is to cross the legs so that the calf of the leg on top is balanced on the knee of the other leg. This is bad for several reasons: first of all, it flattens out the calf and makes the leg look larger. Second, it puts a lot of pressure on the veins in back of the leg, which over a period of time can cause problems with varicose veins and blood vessels. And it's just bad for circulation, in the lower legs particularly.

Another bad thing about crossing your legs is the unconscious tendency to start swinging the leg on top. If you must cross your legs, cross them all the way over so that the calf rests on the side of your knee and leg. Then, slant both legs off to one side. This will give a nice slanted line to your body and make it virtually impossible for you to be swinging the foot. Here again, angle the foot resting on the floor so that it is parallel to the floor. Remember, unconsciously swinging the leg shows nervousness—an annoying mannerism that will weaken your appearance of total confidence.

How do you gracefully get up out of a sitting position?

We will just reverse the procedure. If your legs have been crossed, you will uncross them. Then you move forward to the edge of the chair. One foot should be slightly behind the other to give you better balance as you rise to a standing position without looking down. Simply push with one leg and support the weight of your body with the other as your hands push your body straight up. Remember to push up vertically, never calling attention to your posterior.

There is another sitting position I should touch upon briefly. Many of our casual get-togethers today necessitate sitting on the floor or sitting on steps, or in some other awkward or unusual position. The easiest way is to go down on your knees first—more or less kneel down—and then lean to one side and tuck your legs to one side underneath you. When you get up, reverse the procedure. Get back on your knees and then hope for assistance in rocking back to your feet and standing.

GETTING IN AND OUT OF A CAR

The acid test for graceful movement for women is getting in and out of a car. Is there any graceful way? The basic principles of sitting just outlined will apply with a few adjustments.

To get into the front or back seat of a four-door car gracefully, after the door has been opened for you (or by you), turn so that the back of your calf touches the car. Sit down just as you would sit in a chair. Keep your knees together, and pull your knees and feet into the car in one motion. Follow the same procedure in low sports cars, lifting your legs together to the side, then pulling them into the car.

To get out of the car, keep your knees together, pick up both feet and swing your legs out of the car in one motion. Again, you are reversing movements.

Getting into the back seat of a two-door car is a perplexing problem. Do you back in, tumble in and hope for the best, get halfway in, get stuck and come out to try another way . . . what do you do? Try this the next time you are confronted with this challenge. Hold onto the side of the car for balance and put one foot into the car. (I usually go in with my right foot first.) Bend over from the waist as gracefully as possible, keep your bottom tucked under, pull in the other leg as you sit on the edge of the seat. If necessary to move over for someone else, scoot across the seat; don't walk across half bent over! How do you get out of that predicament? Move back across the seat until you get to the door, keep your knees together (always important), and then extend one foot out the door and push with the other foot. Pull with your hands on the car, or if someone has extended his hand to help, take it. Pulling and pushing, you should manage to get up and out!

The Model's Basic Stance and Pivot

Women are confronted with many different occasions when they have to be photographed full length or simply need to stand properly. We've all seen women standing flat-footed, feet apart, looking very awkward. And we've seen women standing who are models of beauty, poise and loveliness. What made the difference? It's called "the model's basic stance." Any woman can learn to do it.

Place your back foot parallel with your audience, with the heel of the front foot several inches in front of the ball of the back foot. Then you break the ankle of the front foot slightly inward. Keep your weight on the back leg with that knee slightly flexed for balance. The knee of the front leg should also be slightly broken.

The basic model pivot is a three-step process. One: step out always on the foot that is in front; two: bring the back foot around and place it in a parallel position going the other way; three: as you make that turn, bring the other foot back around and gracefully pull it into the correct position in front of the ball of the back foot. When you are ready to complete your turn, follow the same three steps, always stepping out on the foot in front. Practice until you can make a smooth turn in two fluid motions.

If you are asked to model for a local fashion show, this one pivoting step, along with a very graceful carriage and

(Audience is here.)

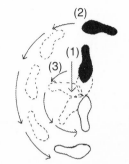

Begin pivot from model's stance, front foot pointed toward audience and back foot parallel to audience (shaded outline). (1) Step forward with front foot, beginning body turn in direction of arrows. (2) Bring back foot around to parallel position in opposite direction, (3) at the same time allowing front foot to pivot 180° on ball of foot. You are now in the model's stance with your back toward the audience (open outline). Practice these movements until you can do them in one fluid motion.

To get back to original position, go through the same movements again. With return to model's stance facing audience, you have completed one full turn.

walk, should take you through most anything. But beyond that, you will have learned how to stand gracefully and comfortably, and how to move from a standing position into action, all with grace and ease.

What Do You Do with Your Hands?

What do you do with your hands when you aren't talking? Hand positions should never become static or fixed, nor rotate in any set way. But in situations that require you to stand and to keep your hands quiet, what can you do with them so as not to appear awkward? Do you cross your arms in front of you like a wooden soldier, or in back of you like a shy schoolchild? No.

There are several things you can do. Remember first of all that keeping elbows held rigidly tight to the sides appears to thicken the waist; but if the arms are properly loose and relaxed in correct body alignment, the elbows will just naturally hang a trifle away from the waist and the body. You might want to cup the back of one hand lightly into the palm of the other a little below the waist or a trifle above it. In this position the back edges of the hands and wrists should be touching the body.

You might wish to interlace your fingers in front of your body, below the waist. Curl the fingers slightly and point them downward, palms facing.

Large-breasted women need always to remember not to cross their arms. If you don't have that problem, then you can cross the lower part of your arms well above the waist, actually just below or on a line with the bust. Slant the fingers of each hand up along the inner side of the upper portion of the opposite arm. Keep your fingers relaxed, however, so they will be slightly separate and allow them to curve easily about the arm; do not clutch the arm. And tuck your thumbs under the arm.

The T-square arm position is another possibility. One elbow is bent and the arm extended across the body; the elbow of the other arm is then cupped lightly in the palm. What about placing your hands in a pocket? Permissible, with the thumb outside the pocket, not jamming the hands into the pocket but placing them there lightly and with grace. Never use smoking as an excuse to have something to do with your hands. It's an unsightly crutch!

IN SUMMARY

The winners of the Miss America Beauty Pageants always have beautiful carriage and movement. Their body alignment, the way they walk, sit and stand projects that graceful image which we have come to expect and associate with this coveted title. But the successful contestants do not acquire their skills overnight. These are young women who have brought themselves and their bodies into control through long hours of self-analysis and self-discipline, and who have trained with as much intensity as an athlete. You can achieve this too, with practice and persistence.

Throughout life, the picture of yourself with good carriage, good body alignment, and a graceful walk is a valuable asset. Life is a constant selling process. Whether you are selling yourself to a teacher in school, to a prospective employer, a potential mate, to new friends, you are being judged from that initial meeting and how you are handling yourself. Never mind that someone may be holding a well-written resume about you in their hands; from the very moment you walk in the door, he or she will be making value judgments about you based upon the impression you create even before you begin speaking. Being able to handle yourself confidently, whatever the circumstances, results from a sense of preparedness on your part. Coming off well, visually speaking, will depend upon honest self-appraisal in your life plus your determination to change and or improve in whatever areas need such improvement and change.

Have friends or family members whose opinion you value work with you and give constructive criticism where necessary. That term—constructive criticism—may need some defining. Throughout my life, I have had to recognize that I do have weak areas and to take stock of them. This has been particularly necessary in entering various competitions. Preparing to meet these tough contenders, I have had to sit down with a piece of paper and say to myself, Donna, these are your strong areas, *but these are your weak areas.* I've had to discipline myself to look critically at myself and ask opinions of other people.

If you are thinking, "Well, nobody likes to be criticized," remember that there are two ways of looking at criticism. Constructive criticism given to point out areas where we need improvement or strengthening can be very valuable. Learn to accept this kind of criticism from those whose opinions you value; then you can, I think, actively start working towards the development of those weak areas, strengthening them and overcoming some problems. Negative criticism, on the other hand, given only to hurt you, can put you on the defensive. It is often tricky to discern the spirit in which criticism is made. But it is important nonetheless to be able to recognize constructive criticism, evaluate and apply it.

There is a price to pay for achievement whether in the field of beauty or any vocation or avocation. Sometimes we think of other people as possessing more talent, more beauty, or more knowledge than we. The truth is, however, that the accomplished individuals have simply harnessed their ambitions to their energy and then worked and worked and worked some more to achieve their goals. I have a writer friend who says, "Donna, success comes by aspiration, inspiration and perspiration."

The Apostle Paul says, "In a race, everyone runs but only one person gets first prize. So run your race to win. To win the contest you must deny yourself many things that would keep you from doing your best. An athlete goes to all this trouble just to win a blue ribbon or a silver cup, but we do it for a heavenly reward that never disappears. So I run straight to the goal with purpose in every step. I fight to win. I'm not just shadow-boxing or playing around. Like an athlete I punish my body, treating it roughly, training it to do what it should, not what it wants to. Otherwise I fear that after enlisting others for the race, I myself might be declared unfit and ordered to stand aside" (1 Cor. 9:24–27, TLB).

In succeeding chapters we'll look at other areas of our life in which we need to discipline ourselves. It's great to have purpose in every step. Remember as you work to improve your body alignment, your carriage, the way you walk, sit and stand, that all facets of charm and beauty are interdependent. The most carefully chosen wardrobe cannot do you justice unless displayed with grace of body; a lovely face and beautifully groomed hair can only be appreciated if poised above a beautifully erect body. Practice these posture and movement tips until they become a very natural part of you.

2

Diet, Nutrition, and Physical Fitness

Overheard in a beauty salon: "This world is made up of people who either have too much or not enough of most everything." Think about that for just a moment; it's a rather startling statement. *Too much, or not enough*—is there no in-between?

Have you ever looked at the paintings of the Renaissance era—the heavy women, very large and soft-looking, but with rolls of fat? This was Rembrandt's portrayal of the beauty of his time.

But ideas of beauty vary from culture to culture. We're living in an age where thin is in. It's virtually impossible to pick up a magazine or newspaper these days that isn't focusing upon the damaging effects—both psychologically and physiologically—of being overweight. Hints and helps for weight reduction and maintenance abound.

I find it most enlightening, however, to discover that Walter Trobisch, internationally known counselor, lecturer, and writer, maintains that women who possess a poor self-image, display two symptoms that occur repeatedly: either these women eat too much or they eat too little. Both over-eating and undernourishing one's self are expressions of the same disease—lack of self-love.

If this is true—and I believe Trobisch in his interviews

and studies is confirming what other researchers, psychologists, and analysts now believe—then whether you "have too much or not enough" may warn you of a basic problem that needs attention. Trobisch explains that lack of self-love creates an empty hole. Overeating is the futile attempt of an individual to fill up this empty hole.

But what about undereating, you ask. Undereating, or denying the body what it needs, may cover up an attempt to punish and deny the unloved self. This is another way of saying, "I'd like to get rid of myself, be free of myself."

Either effort is unacceptable behavior. But there is an in-between—the path of self-acceptance and self-love. True, it will demand effort on your part; but the rewards both for yourself and others will be worth everything it's going to cost you in terms of keeping your goal in sight and straining to reach it. Whether you are interested in becoming another Miss America or want to find a husband or to please the one you already have; whether you need to rid yourself of "too much" or feel you don't have "enough" and need more—whatever your reason and your situation, there is help and there is hope.

WHAT IS YOUR MOTIVATION?

Would you believe that I actually began entering beauty pageants because I had an inferiority complex about being skinny? I've always had a complex about my weight. I can remember excruciating periods in my life when I felt like a scarecrow, especially in junior high school. I not only felt that way, but what was worse, I was certain I looked like one! I was mortified to have to dress out for gym because my legs were toothpicks, and my hips—well, they simply didn't exist.

I entered high school with the same problem. I definitely didn't have what the boys would call "a figure"! This was at the time when Bermuda shorts were popular—these were shorts that hit about two or three inches above the knee. I remember the first pair that I got. I wore knee socks with them, and I was thankful for those knee socks because they covered up a lot of my legs. But there wasn't anything I could do about my skinny knees. I knew that in a straight skirt I looked like a stick, so in order to give myself some sort of shape, I used to wear my Bermuda shorts (which were corduroy) underneath my straight skirts. About all this did was to make me look as if I weighed 98 instead of 97!

It may come as a surprise to those readers who have never been underweight to discover what a problem it is. I tried every weight-gaining product that was ever advertised. Nothing worked. But I was determined to lick this thing. I actually began entering pageants to prove to myself that I was as attractive as my schoolmates, to improve my feeling of self-worth.

I entered my first pageant when I was sixteen, a senior in high school. I chose the Miss Union County pageant for obvious reasons—swimsuit competition was not required. There were fifty-three contestants and with my straight hips concealed by a full-skirted party dress, I won! (I did have good carriage.) My high school classmates were still skeptical: "Well, ho-ho, your daddy is a banker and the whole thing was rigged—" That wasn't true, of course. But that challenge was the beginning of things for me, and I was determined then and there to overcome my inferiority feelings about being so skinny. I graduated from high school weighing about 110 pounds at my present height of 5′ 6½″. I was selected a class favorite, but didn't make the finals for Most Beautiful.

I went off to the University of Arkansas knowing full well that if I ever entered any more beauty pageants that I'd have to eat, eat, eat; take vitamins every day; and just be sure that I got enough food and rest. My weight increased maybe two or three pounds by the end of my freshman year in 1960. During that summer, friends encouraged me to enter the Miss Arkansas Pageant. Against my better judgment I entered because I was flattered and still seeking to prove myself. I was 112 pounds at the time and swimsuit competition was 25 percent of the judging. I did not win a preliminary but finished as third runner-up—disappointed, but even more determined.

I took a long, hard, critical look at myself at that point.

I knew I lacked something in several vital areas, and would have to improve before I could ever win the title. Every girl who enters something and loses, if she has any kind of spirit of competition, reacts the same way: losing makes you sit up, take stock and fight harder.

It was time to embark on a carefully calculated self-improvement program. I decided what needed to be done over the next three years if I was to enter that competition again. Of course, high on the priority list was gaining more weight and developing my figure, my legs, and also my talent and poise.

The spring of my sophomore year, my sorority, Delta Delta Delta, nominated me as their candidate for the Miss University of Arkansas title. I didn't use my head. I should have said no, I'm not ready, but I didn't. I ate voraciously for weeks and lost five pounds the week of the pageant because of nerves and busy schedules. The outcome—second runner-up! I had lost again! In a conversation with my steady boyfriend, Tommy—famous last words—I told him, "That's it. It's over; never again!" That didn't last long.

The summer of my junior year I entered another pageant —this time the Arkansas Forestry Queen contest. No swimsuit competition! The judging was based 50 percent on the ability to speak, along with poise, personality and beauty. This was a state title, and I went through the various districts of competition, winning it all the way. Finally I was a winner!

The next year proved to be my most valuable preparation for reentry into the Arkansas Pageant. I spent it out of college touring Arkansas and eleven other states as an ambassadoress for the forest industry (which was the number one industry in the state). I gave 252 speeches on the uses of wood, and how honored I was when the late Senator John McClellan (D-Ark.) heard my speech and asked for a copy. He later entered it into the Congressional Record. I sang at almost every appearance. The year helped my figure too. I was on what I called the "green bean circuit." Green beans and ham or green beans and chicken was a popular menu. Much to my delight, I gained a little weight!

With the year as Arkansas Forestry Queen completed, I

returned to college and continued my efforts to develop my talent, figure, and personality. I was active in a singing group called the U-Arkettes. The summers between my sophomore, junior, and senior years at college I worked in my father's bank earning money for my wardrobe for the Miss Arkansas Pageant.

By the summer of 1963 I knew I was ready—I was twenty-one and a senior at the University of Arkansas. I had worked very hard on my talent presentation; my voice was more mature and I was more mature. I tipped the scales at approximately 120 pounds by that time. It had taken me three years to gain ten pounds! My figure had improved considerably. With renewed determination I entered the competition.

The very first night was swimsuit competition, my weakest area. My chaperone, Mrs. Sue Mason, said, "I'll bet you a quarter that you'll win." I said, "Aha, you're on!" You could have knocked me over with a feather when I won that phase of the competition! At the Miss America Pageant, I was so scared of losing weight that I drank milk shakes and ate fudge brownies in addition to my meals. Imagine my shock and joy when I also won swimsuit competition in Atlantic City as Miss Arkansas! I was fortunate in the Miss Arkansas Pageant the next night to win the talent competition also, so now I was a two-time preliminary winner. (The winner of the third competition—evening gown and interview—is never announced.)

When the judges were tabulating the final ballot, they realized that there was a tie for first place—myself and the girl who became first runner-up. The judges looked at the tally scores again and decided they would go with the young lady who had the most number of points in talent since that was so heavily scored in the Miss America Pageant (50 percent). As it turned out, I had two more points in talent than my first runner-up. Those two points would change my life forever.

I had prepared diligently over those three years to be just perfect in everything. But unknown to me, I was coming off to the judges as being a little bit arrogant. To any girl reading this who might be interested in such competition, I would like to issue this word of caution: there is a very fine line between what appears to be haughtiness and self-confidence and professionalism. It will help to stay on the right side of it if you keep in the back of your mind the word *humility*. (I'll explain more about this and the experience of Miss America in subsequent chapters in the book.)

This chronicle of my struggle with weight problems should convince you that I wasn't born with a perfect figure. So whether you are overweight or underweight, coping with your problem is a battle. Through hard luck and experience, I learned to eat meals and snacks of high nutritional value. I found out that disciplined eating is important not only to maintain my weight, but also to provide the vitality and energy required for a demanding daily schedule. My weight fluctuates now between 123 and 125 pounds, approximately what I weighed when I was Miss America.

Here are the rules I follow for keeping my weight up:
1. Eat often—small, frequent meals and nutritious snacks. This will supply your body with more energy during each day.
2. Eat high calorie, vitamin-rich foods. Choose foods like cheese, ice cream, peanut butter, bread and butter.
3. Take a multiple vitamin tablet daily.
4. Eat the foods you need even though sometimes you do not feel hungry.
5. Get adequate sleep and rest.
6. Drink milk instead of water some of the time when you are thirsty.
7. Avoid drinking large amounts of liquids before or during a meal so that there will be more room for food.

Do remember that good nutrition and disciplined eating habits are equally important for everyone—those who are trying to lose weight, gain weight, maintain their weight and those who have no weight problems. Food not only determines your shape, it also affects the health and beauty of skin, nails, teeth, hair, and eyes. Dark circles under the eyes; sallow complexion; limp, dull hair; clogged pores; frown lines—all are a reflection of poor health habits. An intelligent and informed approach to eating lays the groundwork for health and beauty. It must become a way of life.

I am often asked if I smoke or have ever smoked. Smoking, in my estimation, is a nasty habit that is expensive, dangerous to your health and beauty, and does nothing to add to a woman's attractiveness. I have never smoked, and I believe this is one of the reasons my skin is as good as it is. There is a relationship between skin aging and smoking. It also distresses me to hear women say, "I can't quit smoking because I'll gain weight." They are robbing Peter to pay Paul, as the old saying goes. Obesity and smoking are both bad for your health.

For both health and beauty, choose a wide range of foods within the following basic food groups.

Milk Group	2 8-oz. servings of milk (cheese, ice cream, cottage cheese and yogurt may be used as alternates)
Meat Group	2 2 or 3-oz. servings of meat, fish, poultry, eggs, cheese, or nuts
Vegetables and Fruit	4 or more ½-cup servings (include dark green vegetables, citrus fruits, or tomatoes)
Bread and Cereal	4 or more servings of enriched or whole-grain products (a serving is one slice bread or equivalent amount of cereal, rice or pasta)

The recommended amounts in each food group provide essential nutrients for one day of good eating. The body needs more than 50 nutrients and no vitamin pill can provide them all. Dozens of vitamins must interact for efficient functioning of the body.

To show you the importance of selecting variety as well as quality, here is a list of eight of the most familiar vitamins and the functions they serve, together with their best sources.

VITAMIN A	helps the body resist nose, throat, and eye infections and promotes growth. Sources: apricots, carrots, skim milk, liver and dark green vegetables.

THIAMINE   aids nerve tissues, stimulates appetite, and
                    promotes good muscle tone. Sources: lean
                    meats, fish, and poultry, whole-grain cereals
                    and breads, milk.

RIBOFLAVIN   promotes healthy skin and hair, good diges-
                    tion, and sound nerves. Sources: lean meats,
                    fish, and poultry, eggs, dark-green leafy vege-
                    tables, milk.

VITAMIN B6   aids in synthesis of protein and regulation of
                    the nervous system and helps maintain salt
                    and water balance in the body. Sources: lean
                    meats, whole-grain cereals.

VITAMIN B12   is essential to production of red blood cells
                    and utilization of foods. Sources: beef, liver,
                    oysters, shrimp.

NIACIN   is essential to the normal functioning of the
                    digestive and central nervous system. Sources:
                    meat, fish, green leafy vegetables, whole-grain
                    breads and cereals.

VITAMIN C   promotes healthy gums and skin and increases
                    the body's resistance to infection. Sources:
                    citrus fruits, green leafy vegetables, tomatoes.

VITAMIN D   aids in absorption of calcium and phosphorus.
                    Sources: Vitamin D enriched milk and cereals.

Most dieticians are now agreed that a diet which promotes health and beauty should be high in proteins and
vitamin-rich foods and low in sugar and starch. I also
supplement my diet with protein powder which I mix with
my juice or milk. "Low in starch" does not mean no carbohydrates; everyone needs carbohydrates as a major source
of energy for daily activity. But choose whole-grain breads
and cereals that are not highly sweetened and wholesome
starchy vegetables such as potatoes. Foods should be judged
on the presence and abundance of ingredients essential for
health.

From the many women I have helped in my beauty

classes, I know that more of you are trying to lose weight than gain weight. Choosing from the four food groups in smaller portions is also an excellent idea for a weight control program, but do not expect miracles overnight. Eating for slender beauty requires perseverance, self-discipline, and patience. The safest and most effective way of slimming is to lose weight slowly but steadily. A crash diet can have horrible aging effects on the face and neck and can cause permanent damage to the elasticity of the skin. If you lose large amounts of weight too quickly, your skin will just hang. A slow, well-planned diet has the valuable long-term effect of subtly changing your eating habits. With new patterns of eating, it will be easier to maintain your weight loss once you achieve your ideal weight. The important thing will be, five years from now, how well have you kept the weight off.

Here are the steps that I recommend for sensible weight reduction:

1. See your doctor first. He will check for underlying health problems. He will also prescribe the number of calories for your height and body type and set up a realistic time schedule. Together you can decide on your personal weight goal. The following chart can give you an indication of the range of weight for your height:

DESIRABLE WEIGHTS FOR WOMEN OVER 25

Height (bare feet)		Weight in pounds (in the nude)		
feet	inches	small frame	medium frame	large frame
4	11	95–103	100–112	108–124
5	0	98–106	103–115	111–127
5	1	100–108	105–117	113–129
5	2	103–111	108–121	116–133
5	3	106–114	111–125	120–137
5	4	109–118	115–130	124–141
5	5	113–122	119–134	128–145
5	6	116–125	122–137	131–148
5	7	120–129	126–141	135–152
5	8	124–134	130–145	139–157
5	9	128–138	134–149	143–162
5	10	132–142	138–153	147–167

2. Begin a food diary. Write down every single thing you eat each day and total up the number of calories. Measure everything, using teaspoons, tablespoons, ounces, or other descriptive measures. What you want is a reasonable estimate of your usual daily food intake. Your eating habits may differ at different times of the day and on certain days of the week and month. Progress will depend on how well you keep your food record. If your weight loss is unsatisfactory, look for negative eating patterns that will emerge after the diary is kept for several weeks.

3. Eliminate foods of low nutritional value. Check this list for possible sources of extra, no- or low-vitamin calories:

> sugar, candy, syrup
> jelly, preserves
> cakes, cookies, pies
> pastries, sweet rolls
> gravies, rich sauces
> heavy salad dressings
> whipped toppings
> popcorn, potato chips
> doughnuts, fried snacks
> sweetened soft drinks
> alcoholic beverages

4. Eat breakfast. Your body has fasted all night and needs the energy boost of a morning meal. Breakfast will get you through the day with less snacking and more energy. I always eat breakfast.

5. Keep meals and snacks enjoyable. Make eating a special occasion by using a pretty placemat and cloth napkin. Serve the food attractively on your best china, selecting a small plate if portions look miserly. Put away your reading materials and turn off the television. Enjoy, enjoy, enjoy. Savor every bite. Become aware of the wonderful variety in foods—colors, flavors, and textures.

6. Begin an exercise program. Exercise alone won't accomplish a major weight loss, but even an additional thirty minutes a day can add up over weeks and months to a significant caloric expenditure. Exercise also contributes to a lithe, well-proportioned body and a general sense of well-

being. With exercise, you'll be amazed how much better you will feel about yourself and your body.

7. Drink lots of water. Calorie-free water fills the stomach and decreases appetite. It also facilitates the excretion of waste materials from the body and generally cleanses the system of impurities. Excessive coffee and tea and diet cola drinks lead to jangled nerves, complexion problems, and poor digestion. It is the caffeine in these drinks that causes problems.

8. Never eat fast. Take plenty of time and chew your food well. It takes thirty to forty-five minutes, from the first mouthful of a meal, for your blood sugar to rise to the point where you no longer feel hungry. Devoting forty-five minutes to a meal is a method any woman can use to keep herself slim. (It can also give a family time to communicate with each other.)

With these principles in mind, try this sample menu. The foods suggested are tasty and nutritious as well as beneficial to your weight-loss program. Remember, this menu is only a guide; there are many delicious alternatives.

BREAKFAST

Half a grapefruit
One egg
One slice toast
One teaspoon butter
Milk

LUNCH

Chicken salad made with
One teaspoon mayonnaise
One slice rye toast
Lettuce and celery sticks
½ banana or small pear
Milk

DINNER

4-oz. broiled steak
Cauliflower
Broccoli spears
Romaine lettuce salad with
One teaspoon oil, plus vinegar
One slice whole-grain bread

Following this kind of sensible diet allows you to eat
quite normally and to sit at the table with your family.
You'll lose weight, but you will also gain in energy and a
sense of well-being.

Exercise Your Way to Fitness and Health!

I have never liked exercising just for the sake of exercising. I would be less than honest if I didn't tell you that. I
am not that great on sports either. How then do I keep myself limber and maintain muscle tone? I learned long ago
that there are some things we make ourselves do even
though we don't feel like it. I have found out that when
I am under a lot of stress and haven't taken care of my body
—if I haven't eaten properly, taken my vitamins, haven't
received enough rest, *and* haven't exercised—that my body
just won't work for me. So I do my toning exercises for
20–30 minutes a day as I'm watching TV or listening to my
favorite snappy music.

As Miss America I had to make it through 365 strenuous
days my reigning year. My daily routine had to allow me to
accomplish all that was required and provide me with a
good balance of physical energy and also that vitality so
necessary to be a sparkling Miss America. I learned then
that exercise is essential, and that basic fact is still with me.

Exercise goes hand in hand with dieting. Not only are
you burning up calories, but you are keeping your body in
good working order and developing your heart (which is a
muscle), and you are keeping the blood circulating which
in turn keeps the skin looking healthy and keeps the impurities out. Everything works together in your best interests.

Here are the exercises which I find enjoyable and relaxing,
and they do the job. *Remember*—take all exercises slowly
and gradually build up to a routine.

    I. Waistline, upper hips.
        A. Standing stretch.
            Stretch up to the ceiling. Try to touch it with one
            hand, then the other. Stretch so that the rib cage
            moves up. Relax-bounce to the floor—don't strain!

B. Side stretch.

Legs apart, hips tucked under, hands to side, stretch to the right with the left arm. Follow with the rest of the body. Bounce four times to the right side; raise right arm and *stretch* 4 times to the left. Repeat 10 times.

C. Floor touch.

Legs apart, arms above head, turn to the right and touch the outside of the right foot. Bounce and touch between your legs; bounce and touch to the left. Repeat 5 times to the right and 5 times to the left.

II. Neck (great to relieve tension in the neck and for general relaxation).

A. Head roll.

Sit on the floor, legs crossed, hands on knees. Slowly roll head to the right shoulder, down to the chest, then to the back. Continue to circle with a slow, relaxed motion. Do 4 to the left, 4 to the right.

B. Double chin stretch.

Let your head drop back. Open your mouth; then close it. Stretching the jaw upward, slowly lift head as if pulling it by the top of your ears, away from your shoulders to the starting position.

III. Inner thigh.

A. Leg bounce.

Sit in an upright, cross-legged position, back straight. Bend your knees out and clasp your feet in front of you. Bounce knees up and down.

B. Inner leg stretch.

Still in seated position, spread your legs apart. Bending from the waist, extend arms toward toes; stretch to the left leg. Do 5 each direction.

C. Exercises to strengthen the back muscles.

1. Lean forward from the waist, extending both arms straight in front of you, and reach—really stretch. Bounce and extend some 15–20 times.

2. The leg thrust—balance your weight on both hands and one knee. Now lower your head as

you bring the other knee up to your chin. Arch
your back and extend the leg backward and up.
Repeat 10–15 times; then change legs. Also
good for stomach muscles.

IV. Hips.
 A. Leg raise I.
   Lie on your side, raise leg parallel to the floor, foot
   flexed and parallel. 15 times on each side.
 B. Leg raise II.
   Lie on your side, head resting on outstretched
   arm. Keep legs straight; point toes. Keep legs together and raise them off the floor 2 inches. Hold.
   Raise 2 inches more. Hold. Lower legs to the floor
   and relax. Do 5 times; reverse.
 C. Stand erect on the toes of one foot while holding
   onto a chair. Swing other leg backwards at a 90°
   angle. Repeat 20 times. You will feel the action in
   the fanny muscles. Helps maintain a firm rounded
   appearance.

V. Outside of thighs.
 A. Lie on your side with head resting on outstretched
   arm. Raise your top leg; raise bottom leg to touch
   top leg; lower bottom leg; lower top leg. Do 8
   times on each side.
 B. "Fire hydrant."
   Get down on your hands and knees. Raise left leg
   to the side parallel to the floor. Knees bent, extend
   leg *slowly* and hold. Do 5 times on each side.

VI. Calves (to build up only).
 A. Stand with the ball and toes of one foot resting
   on a step or thick book. Raise and lower body 20
   times on each leg.

VII. Abdomen.
 A. Situps.
   Remember—knees always bent, feet flat on the
   floor. Gradually increase number of repetitions.

VIII. Waist and hips.
 A. Knee and chest roll.
   Lie on your back, arms extended to the side. Pull
   knees to the chest; roll knees to the right elbow;

bring them to the chest again and roll to the left elbow. Work up to 20 repetitions daily.
  B. Stand with feet apart and extend your arms to the front. Swing them as far as you can to each side.
IX. Arms.
  A. Isometric push.
     Lie on back, arms close to the body, palms outstretched on the floor. Push hard 5 times. Now clench your fists and press hard to the floor 5 times.
 X. Bust (this exercise will build up the pectoral muscles which support the breast—giving beautiful bustline).
  1. Lie on your back with arms extended straight out from your side. Using a book or weight in each hand, raise and lower arms, meeting over your head. Repeat 20 times.
  2. Wall push-ups.
     Place feet about 1½ to 2 feet from a wall. Extend your arms and push your body away from the wall. Repeat 20 times.
  3. Arm circles.
     Extend your arms straight out from your side. Move your arms in small circles, first forward, then backward. Repeat 20 times each way.

In Summary

I discovered in my development classes, and in talking to women across the country, that many women's problems result from boredom. They are bored with themselves and life in general. I realize, too, that more women have problems losing weight than putting weight on. What many fail to realize is that a weight gain didn't come about overnight and neither will a weight loss. Don't expect miracles; those ten, twenty, thirty, or more pounds aren't going to come off in a couple of weeks. It doesn't happen that way.

Remind yourself that anything worthwhile takes time and work, dedication and determination. Set a weight goal; be persistent and have a source of motivation. It took me four years of self-discipline, with setbacks and disappointments many times along the way, before that Miss America crown was placed on my head. It also took me four years to gain twelve valuable pounds.

The book of Ecclesiastes contains some choice wisdom. Think about these verses as you take yourself in hand and set about to reach some desired goals: "Finishing is better than starting! Patience is better than pride!" (7:8, TLB). "Tackle every task that comes along, and if you fear God you can expect his blessing" (7:18, TLB).

❧ 3 ❧

Skin Care and Makeup

God is the Master Designer. He created you and made you a unique individual, a "Designer creation," not exactly like anyone else on this earth. You may not like every feature, but the fact remains, you are what you are. What you do with your potential is what is important. Unlike yesteryear, today we have no set, strict definition of beauty. We don't have to try to fashion ourselves after Marilyn Monroe or Elizabeth Taylor, for natural beauty in a variety of looks is today's theme. So accept yourself. Be happy with what is you and learn to enhance the beauty of the outer you with good skin care and makeup skills.

PREVENTIVE SKIN CARE

Beautiful skin is one of woman's most treasured possessions. Millions of dollars are spent each year in America on cosmetic and skin care products. Even the most expensive products, however, will not insure good skin. There are a number of elements that affect the final result. Let's take a look at them, as they are an integral part of the finished product.

Heredity and Health

The two factors of heredity and health alone are the basis of skin care and maintenance. Skin type is determined at conception—fair or dark, oily or dry, sensitive or coarse, or other variations. This we cannot change—we can only learn to work with what we have. Generally, health, stress, emotional or physical problems, and allergies all have major effects on the skin. Female problems, hormone imbalance, surgery—all these factors register on our skin and can often serve as a warning to us of physical problems. We have already discussed how important exercise, rest and plenty of water are in keeping our skin in beautiful healthy condition.

Environment

The sun is our number one enemy from two standpoints. Overexposure to its rays can cause skin cancer, and it also causes premature aging and wrinkling, sun spots and broken capillaries. Formerly it was considered very fashionable and healthy-looking to sport a tan. But is it really worth it in the long run to look older than your years, hard and leathery? Is it worth the risk of skin cancer?

If you do spend some time in the sun, learn to protect your skin from its drying effects with hats, protective screening lotions, and good common sense. Don't overexpose your skin. Bad sunburns can cause permanent damage. Dermatologists also tell me that the tanning lotions that tan without the sun are not harmful and are far better for your skin than the sun. Wind, salt water, and air pollution all have harmful effects. Protect your skin from these elements. You will be rewarded with more beautiful, younger looking skin.

One more harmful element should be mentioned here, and I consider it a major one—smoking. It causes the skin to age more rapidly and take on a shallow yellowish cast. Not only is this habit harmful to your health, but it is most detrimental to your skin beauty and femininity. In short—don't smoke!

Start Early and Stick With It

While I was Miss America, the demands made upon my time were unbelievably strenuous. With sixteen-hour days not uncommon, I discovered at the outset that I would really have to take care of myself. Subjecting the body to continual stress and strain inevitably takes a toll. So a disciplined life then became a matter of necessity, and continues to be to this day as I still maintain a strenuous schedule.

Even the best skin care program won't do it all from the outside. We know the human body is an interacting system. The skin is a living organ of the body, our largest organ. Doesn't it make sense that the better your health, the better will be your skin? Protect what you have by practicing a preventive skin care program. The dividends will be multifaceted. Be good to yourself and you'll notice the difference in beautiful, healthy-looking skin within weeks. The secret to beautiful skin really is more than just skin deep.

It is vitally important to begin caring for the skin at an early age, as early as the pre-teen years, and to continue on a regular, regimented program. Why? Because the finished product is no better than the skin you start with. This preventive step helps you look better longer. If you are beyond the "early age" phase of your life, start where you are now. You cannot totally reverse the damage, but you can improve your skin and slow down the aging process.

Skin Types

The first step in establishing a skin care program is to determine your skin type—normal, dry, oily, or a combination of any of these. Generally, it's pretty easy to decide, but if you have any difficulty, consult a trained cosmetic representative at one of your local stores. How you clean and care for your skin, as well as the types of makeup you select, will depend on your skin type. This is especially important if you have sensitive, allergic, or problem skin. See a dermatologist immediately to help identify any problems that occur and to prevent permanent scarring.

Every year the major cosmetic houses introduce new and better products. Watch the cosmetic counters in your favorite department and drug stores and sample some of these products from time to time. I have found it best to stick with the same brand in both skin care and cosmetic lines as they are chemically balanced to work together to produce the best results. Once you have found dermatologist-tested and approved products that work well for you, stick with them, but do keep up with what's current, and make a change if you find a clearly better product.

If your skin is normal to oily, use a mild soap, face wash, or medicated wash as recommended by your doctor. Follow with an astringent and, if needed, a moisture lotion. Everyone, regardless of skin type, needs a moisturizer and night cream around the eyes. This area is a number one target for aging, so be careful.

Dry Skin

If you have dry skin, try not to use soap on your face as it has a very drying effect. In fact, use only very mild defatted soaps when you bathe—never harsh detergent soaps. Clean your face with cleansing cream or a mild face wash. Remove the cleansing agent with a clean soft rag or tissue. Rinse your face frequently with water to plump up the cells. Stay away from extremely hot water—warm to temperate water is recommended for bathing as it is not as great a shock to the skin. In addition, remember that bathing too frequently continuously robs the skin of its precious oil. If your skin is extremely dry, try total bathing every other day and sponge washing in between.

Normal Skin

If you are blessed with normal skin—congratulations. This means that you will have fewer problems to cope with over the years. A good, basic skin care program is all with which you will have to be concerned. Don't be overconfident and neglect your skin. Instead, treat it as the precious possession that it is. You will be able to choose from a wide variety of makeup and skin care products, selecting those that work best for you. You may clean your face with a mild skin soap, face wash, or cleansing cream. Always follow with an astringent and moisturizer. A heavier use of cream around the eyes at night is always good.

Oily Skin

If oily skin is yours, then you are constantly plagued with the problems of clogged pores and blemishes and a tendency toward blackheads and whiteheads. And from a purely esthetic standpoint, it's hard to look fresh and lovely if your face is shiny ten minutes after you have applied your makeup. You will have to be especially careful to avoid acne by following a good skin care routine. If acne does become a problem, see a dermatologist immediately to help minimize permanent scarring. Although acne is usually a teenage problem, dermatologists are seeing more and more adult acne caused by stress and other physical factors. So you're never too old to have it.

It is especially important that you keep your skin as clean as possible at all times to help minimize skin problems. Wash your face at least twice a day, or as frequently as you can within the framework of your daily routine. A drying soap with water or a dermatologist-recommended facial wash is ideal. Once again, everyone has special needs, so experiment until you find what is right for you. Following your cleansing, apply an astringent for oily skin with a cotton pad. This removes all traces of makeup and oil and tightens your pores. Apply a moisturizer around the eye area only. Remember, too, that it is especially important for you to drink plenty of water to keep skin impurities flushed out of your pores. Here is another pointer—don't use powder to cover the shine on your face. This will only compound your problems in the long run as you constantly add more powder on top of makeup, oil, and dirt, clogging your pores even more. You also risk transferring more bacteria from a dirty puff. Instead of powder, try face savers—individual sheets of absorbent tissue that will remove the oil.

Combination Skin

A large percentage of women have what is known as combination skin—a combination of normal skin with oily areas or dry skin with oily areas. The oily areas are usually in a T-shaped area across the forehead, nose, and chin. It's important to remember that you have to treat each area differently in your skin care program. Use the products appropriate for each type of skin.

MASKS

Treat yourself to the total cleansing of a facial mask at least once a week. The purpose of a mask is to draw to the surface the dirt and oil that clog the pores. It also assists in removing the layer of dead skin cells that are constantly being sluffed off by our bodies, and it stimulates the circulation. During this facial, lie back, put your feet up, and try relaxing every muscle in your body, including facial muscles. It is a great lift. Once again, the frequency and type of product used is dependent on your skin type.

MOISTURIZERS

Water and moisture are, in my opinion, the two most important ingredients in maintaining soft, radiant skin. Water taken internally—six to eight glasses per day—and water used externally keep the skin cells soft and full. When our skin loses vital moisture it dries out, peels, and shows aging lines. Moisturizers protect the skin by helping it retain that vital water. Again the type and frequency of use of a moisturizer will depend upon your skin type, but it is essential for most skins. This is especially true around the eye area. There are no oil glands there and the skin is very thin and susceptible to dryness. Gently work creams and lotions in this area, using the third finger, as it has less force. Work from the outer corner of the eye, using a light patting motion. Never stretch the skin and be very careful when removing eye makeup. Cotton and a mascara remover are most desirable. Baby oil is an economical second choice. Use an upward motion for removal rather than pulling down on the delicate skin around the eyes.

I use a moisturizer at least twice a day—once in the morning before applying my makeup and again at night after cleansing. Heavier eye creams are effective around the eyes area at night while you sleep.

Don't Scrub and Rub

We've all heard of "the well scrubbed look." It's good to have clean skin, but bad to achieve it by rubbing and scrubbing. Here's why. We are born with a great amount of elasticity in our skin. But as we grow older and subject our skin to all the various elements, it looses that elasticity and begins to sag—thus the bags under the eyes the jowls at the jaw and neckline. It is important, therefore, as we clean our face or apply makeup to do so gently and in an upward motion.

Follow the directions of the arrows in this illustration, always an upward motion.

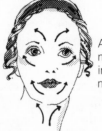

Always apply makeup or creams in an upward motion

When applying creams or makeup, use the third finger instead of the middle one as it has less strength and is more gentle on the skin.

Avoid scrubbing your face with a cloth or coarse facial tissues. Gently wipe, always in an upward motion.

Here's a final thought to remember. It is important to keep your skin as clean as possible to let your skin breathe and avoid skin problems. Never go to bed with dirty skin or makeup on regardless of how tired you are. Keep it clean and let your skin rest as you sleep. Don't forget to clean it again in the morning. Even while you were asleep, your body was still pumping out oils and impurities. Also, on the weekends as I'm doing my housework, I'll give myself a long pampering facial and leave off makeup so my skin can rest.

CHOOSING THE RIGHT MAKEUP

Makeup styles, like fashion, change from year to year, and it is imperative that you keep your look updated. Don't ever be guilty of combining current fashions with a dated look in makeup. It's very easy to become comfortable with a look. Just because you looked great in it ten years ago doesn't mean that you'll turn heads with it today. Usually it is a dead giveaway of the year you graduated from high school or college. Stay in the know, keep updated, and you will reflect the self-confidence you feel. You can best do this by watching the fashion magazines and beauty guides and by observing other attractive and fashionable women. Don't be afraid to experiment.

Over the years, whenever I've seen a particularly striking woman, I've studied her closely. If I have an opportunity to get up close to her, while I'm talking to her I try to analyze how she achieved her certain look. I do the same thing with models in magazines. The next time you see a photograph of a beautiful woman in a fashion or beauty magazine, go a step further—look closely and break the beautiful look down into minute areas (in particular if it's a closeup of the individual's face). Concentrate, for instance, on where she put eye shadow, or what colors she mixed to achieve the particular look she had created. Then try to recreate that look for your particular coloring and facial features if it is appropriate for you. One word of caution: the dramatic effects of high fashion makeup can be overpowering in everyday life. Tone it down.

My first suggestion is to visit a reputable cosmetic counter in a store that has a good variety of cosmetic lines and talk with the various representatives. Often someone there will even demonstrate their products to you, and from time to time the manufacturers also send representatives for the same purpose. If you have sensitive skin, you will want to be particularly careful in selecting hypoallergenic makeup and skin care products. Cosmetics are an investment, and costly mistakes can be avoided with some prudent shopping. Take the necessary time before buying. As you shop you will notice a wide range in prices. There is usually a satisfactory product for your price range.

I think that it is important before making any major purchases to decide how you want your makeup to relate to your lifestyle as it enhances your natural beauty. Only you can make that decision. Let me share my two basic philosophies with you: (1) the finished product (the made-up face) is no better than the skin you start with, so give it tender loving care; (2) it is not how much makeup you can apply that is important but how little to achieve the natural, glowing, desired results. In other words, don't mask your beauty with heavy clownlike makeup; instead, develop your makeup expertise so that you learn to enhance your face through the art of color and contouring, blended to perfection.

MAKEUP BASE

The purpose of a foundation is to give your face an even tone and to cover any blemishes or problem areas. It is the prime base for the entire effect. It is important to select the right type of makeup (oil or water base) depending upon your skin type and the correct color. Water-based foundations are for young and oily skins, oil-based for dry skin. The consistency will usually determine the degree of coverage. Lotions provide a light cover and pan stick, creams, and cake the most coverage. I recommend the latter for on-stage work, such as speaking, performing, pageants, and similar needs. A word of caution again: apply the foundation a little at a time and blend it thoroughly. You can always add more if you need it, but if it's too thick from the beginning you will have to start over.

The color selection should be as close to your natural skin color as possible. (Remember to use a darker base in the summer when you tan). Test for color on your jawbone, blending the sample down your neck slightly. This is a far truer test than on your wrist.

Apply and blend the base on one part of the face at a time. Remember to use a gentle upward motion. Carry the base under your jaw and chin line just slightly and a little down your neck. Avoid a line that stops at the jaw. I do not extend the makeup down the neck. It is not necessary and is very difficult to remove from clothing. An under-eye cover stick can be applied either before or after base applications. I prefer to do it before and to blend the two together. This provides effective cover for dark circles and other blemishes.

Contouring

This subtle art used correctly will turn an ordinary face into a beautiful sculpture. How? By emphasizing bone structure and features.

One basic principle applies in the art of contouring, and that is the principle of light and dark. Pale shades reflect light, causing an area to seem more prominent; the dark shades absorb light, creating a shadow. Thus, if you want to lift into prominence the cheekbones and browbones, you would apply a highlighter, a light foundation—pink or white. If you want your face to appear slimmer, or if you have a broad nose and want to give the effect of diminishing it, then contour with darker shades in those areas. Is there a hint of a double chin? Contour under your jawbone below the chin, and be sure to blend down into the shadow below the chin. Don't be afraid to use a cosmetic for a purpose other than that for which it was intended, for instance, a light brown eyebrow pencil or eye color sticks that are very, very soft work well for contouring.

Some cosmetic companies produce products especially for this purpose. My favorites are the cocoa brown powders that are similar to blushes and applied with a brush.

These illustrations show placement for the basic contouring areas suggesting light and dark.

Always remember this rule: light and shine bring an area forward, while dark makes it less prominent. Work with a light hand and blend carefully.

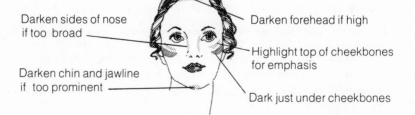

Darken sides of nose if too broad

Darken chin and jawline if too prominent

Darken forehead if high

Highlight top of cheekbones for emphasis

Dark just under cheekbones

BLUSHERS AND ROUGES

One of the finest things that has come along in the cosmetic world in the past twenty years is the blusher. Almost every face needs the lift this touch of color and look of glowing health brings. Apply it a little at a time and blend. A point to remember: apply a greater amount of color if you are going to be on stage or under bright lights, as the lights will make you look washed-out.

If you have a dry skin, a liquid or a cream will blend better, last longer, and look lovelier. If you intend to use a powder blusher, apply it just before powdering. When you apply the cream blusher, go back to the cheekbone area, start at the hairline, and work no further forward than halfway toward your nose. Blend carefully a little bit at a time with a very soft touch so as not to disturb your foundation. If you have done contouring, place the blusher slightly above the contour area and then blend the two together. I find a little dab of blusher just underneath my chin gives my face a lift from below. I have also discovered that a liquid or cream blusher topped by a powder blusher has greater staying power. I apply the liquid or cream first, blending gently; after it has set a bit, I use just a bit of powder blusher to set the other.

Always select a color that blends with your skin tones and is not too harsh for your coloring. This will help you avoid the "clown look" of vivid round circles of color. Remember also that your blusher and lipstick color should be in the

Apply blusher for a more radiant look

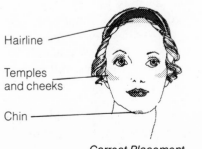
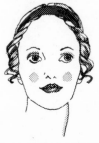

Hairline

Temples and cheeks

Chin

Correct Placement   *Incorrect placement*

same hue-related family. For example, pinks and plums together and reds, apricots, peaches together.

Nothing takes the place of nature's lovely glow but a blusher will add that wonderful look of vitality for a radiant face.

The "Eyes" Have It

Probably no other feature is as important as the eyes, for not only do they allow us to see the beautiful world around us, but they are our most important tool in nonverbal communication. They are indeed the windows of our souls—reflecting every human emotion. It is important, therefore, that they be attractively accentuated.

Let's begin with the framing—the eyebrows. Strive to achieve a natural-looking brow with a curved arch. Be sure to pluck all unnecessary hairs under the brow line. This cleans up the upper lid area and makes the eyes look more open. The start of your brow can be determined by placing 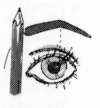 a pencil by the side of your nose and extending it upward. Your natural arch should be just above the outer sides of your iris. Carefully shape your brows with tweezers only. Never shave them; they may not grow back as before. Remember that a natural-looking brow is always in style. Don't be tempted to follow fads in brow styles. Not only can this be dating, but might also cause irreversible damage. If your brows are too light or thin, correct them with a fine-line eyebrow pencil for the most natural look. Make short, hairlike strokes. Avoid a black pencil, as it is too harsh even for women with black hair. A good rule of thumb to follow is one shade lighter than your hair. Please—no heavily drawn-on eyebrows, and don't stop your eye makeup with the brows. Finish the picture with eye shadows and mascara.

Eye Shadowing and Lashes

The purpose of using eye shadow is threefold: (1) to accentuate the color of the eyes; (2) to add definition, thus making them look larger; and (3) for contouring and shape correction purposes.

Today there seems to be no rule of thumb for color selection. I would suggest, however, that regardless of the shade you select that it be subtle enough to accentuate and not dominate. The color should not jump out and grab your attention but should blend into the total eye effect. Eyeshadow should be less intense during the day and a little more dramatic for evening. Although I occasionally wear greens and blues, I prefer a combination of peach or pink and brown. This combination seems to create the best consistent accent for my brown eyes. It is not necessary for your eyeshadow always to match the color of your dress.

The type of shadow that you select—cream or powder—depends to a great degree on your age and skin type. Normal skins can use either. Oily skins should use powder and dry skins cream shadows. Powdered shadows tend to make older or dry skin look crepelike. Also stay away from the frosted or metallic products.

Here are two basic ways of applying eye shadows: (1) using a highlighter and brown combination, and (2) using a color, plus brown for contouring and a browbone highlighter. (Never apply color from lash base to eyebrow; always stop with the color just under the brow bone.)

Women with deep-set eyes should wear lighter shades in order to bring out the eyes. Never use brown or dark colors; they will tend to make the eyes look even more deepset.

Two basic ways to apply eye shadow

(1)

Highlighter just under browbone—pink, peach or light beige—never white

Brown contouring—apply from inner corner outward; blend, placing in hollow of eye under browbone

Highlighter from base of lashes to hollow

(2)

Highlighter

Brown contouring, or lighter colors in darker values

Apply color starting at base of lashes

As you can see, you can use eye shadow not only to complement but also to correct. Just remember the principles of light and dark—light enlarges and advances; dark minimizes and recedes.

Eye Liner

The next step in eye makeup is eye liner. Eye liner comes and goes in fashion history. In the '60s thick black liner was in fashion, but the '70s have seen us go toward a more natural look. You may not want to wear it at all, but if you do, here are a couple of tips.

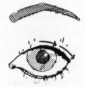

Normal to large eyes.

Apply the liner in a very thin line just at the base of the lashes, starting at the inner corner and extending to the outer corner. Do not extend it past the corner of the eye. This "winged" effect went out in the '60s. You can get the finest line by applying the liner with the tip of the brush rather than the side. Balance your hand by resting your little finger on your cheek. A black eyeliner is too harsh. Choose instead a brown, charcoal, or gray, depending upon your coloring.

Small or Close-set Eyes.

Start your liner about at the middle or three-quarters of the way to the outside. This will make them look larger and more wide-set. (If you have protruding eyes, don't wear liner; it will only add to the problem. Instead, stick to the darker shadows.) Never totally rim your eyes with a dark liner. This will make them look even smaller.

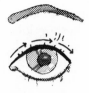

Wide-set Eyes.

To make your eyes seem closer together, apply your eyeshadow in the sideways "v" fashion, as illustrated, and carefully blend. Extend the shadow under the lower lashes and carefully blend.

Before applying the last step, mascara, I lightly dust my eyelids with a translucent powder (use a sable brush) to help set the makeup.

Additional tips:

1. For a more dramatic effect, apply a soft pencil eye liner to the inner rim of your lower lid. Use a dark brown, blue, or green. Again, black is too harsh.

2. For greater definition, I apply a dark brown soft pencil color under my bottom lashes from about the center to the outer edge of the eye. Smudge the line slightly to soften it. You can do the same thing with the color eye shadow that you are using.

"THE ICING ON THE CAKE"

Mascara and Lashes

Certainly, few layer cakes would look complete without the icing. Similarly, the eye makeup is not complete without attention to the lashes. First of all, I think that you ought to take care of your own eyelashes. Eyelashes are hair, and just like the hair on your head, you must take care of them. One of the best things to do, and a precautionary measure, is always to clean your eyelashes every night. They need to be free of mascara so they can breathe. These are hair follicles; if you clog them, they aren't going to breathe naturally, and you may lose them. If you have trouble losing your lashes, you might check the mascara you are using. You might be allergic to it and need to try another kind. Some loss is natural.

Most lashes are longer than they look, as they tend to be lighter on the tip end. Mascara creates miracles by coloring the lash to the end and thickening it in the process. Select black, blackish brown, or brown depending upon your coloring. Black is too harsh for blondes. I prefer an automatic roll-on brush applicator that curls the lashes upward as it colors them.

Apply the mascara by beginning at the base of the lashes and working up. Look straight into the mirror as you apply it, not down. For thicker-looking lashes, apply two or three coats, waiting about thirty seconds between applications. For additional curl, use an eyelash curler before applying your mascara. Be sure the rubber banding on the curler is in good shape and don't push down too hard. To use an eyelash curler, look straight into the mirror and place the curler as close to the base of the lashes as possible. Close and hold it for about ten seconds. Carefully open and remove it. If you don't catch the lash at the base you come up with a "fish hook" look.

You can thicken the lashes by lightly dusting the lashes with powder and then adding a second coat. Please don't overdo this. Nothing looks worse than thick gloppy-looking lashes.

Apply mascara also to your lower lashes. Now the total eye is complete. Remember: the key words are accent, contour and color.

False Lashes

Unless you really don't have any lashes of your own, I advise you not to wear false eyelashes. Soon the wear and tear they do to your own lashes will make you totally dependent on them on a full-time basis. Also, it takes real skill and practice to be able to select, trim and apply false lashes so as to make them appear natural.

There are special times, however, that you may feel the need to wear them, such as for photography or stage presentations or for evening wear. If so, here are a few tips to follow:

1. Select the type that best suits your particular need according to the thickness of your own lashes and the size of your eyes. You will be able to select from a demi-lash (half-lash width and usually shorter in lash length also) to the full, long, extra-thick lash. Make your color selection based on your hair color.

2. Don't wear the lashes straight out of the box. Measure them to your own eye width and trim them accordingly, from the outer edge. If you feel that they are too long for your taste, shorten them by careful trimming. Never cut them straight across. Instead, cut each lash by clipping toward the band, staggering the lash lengths slightly as you go. The lashes toward the inner corner of the eye should be shorter than the outer corner.

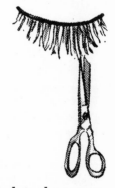

Now you are ready for application. This takes some skill and practice. First mascara your own lashes; they will stick together better with the false lashes and give a more unified look. Next pick up the lash in the center, using an eyebrow tweezer. Carefully apply the adhesive on the very top of the band, not the side. Be careful not to get too much. Now let the adhesive set for about ten seconds before applying to the eye.

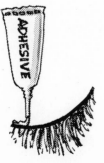

(You may apply it straight out of the tube or place it on a toothpick and spread it across)

Looking straight into the mirror, place the lash on the center position of your eyelid. Make sure that it is as close to the base of your own eyelid as possible. Now hold

Applying false eyelashes

Right   Wrong

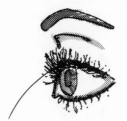   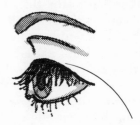

Lashes should rest on edge   You should not be able to look at
                                the eye and see the top of the
                                band

it in position for about ten to fifteen seconds. Release the tweezers carefully and grasp the outer lash. Press it into place and hold it until it slightly dries. Repeat the same process for the inner corner of the eye. Before the lash dries completely, take your fingers and press the false lash and your own together to avoid a separation. Tilt the false lash up for a more wide open look. The lash should adhere by the top of the band rather than the inside.

If the lash comes unglued, place some adhesive on a toothpick and carefully repair it.

You may want to add additional mascara as a final touch.

Lower lashes look extremely fake to me and I do not recommend them.

To remove the lashes, carefully pull from the outside corner in. After each wearing, remove the dried adhesive. From time to time you will want to remove the built-up mascara by cleaning the lashes. Wash them in a liquid soap and water. Curl them around a pencil to dry. This should establish their shape again.

If your eyes get allergic to the adhesives that come with the lashes, or if they turn red after wearing the lashes for only a few minutes, try a surgical adhesive instead. This usually eliminates the problem. If it doesn't, don't wear the lashes for long periods of time or not at all. It's really not worth the eye irritation.

THE MOUTH—IT SPEAKS FOR ITSELF

After the eyes, the mouth is the most expressive feature of the face. A beautiful mouth and lovely smile can be your most valuable asset as it communicates verbally and nonverbally the beautiful inner you. All Miss Americas do not look alike, but do share one similar characteristic—a beautiful smile. Here is how to perfect a beautiful mouth and smile with care, color, and shine.

Oral Hygiene

Any discussion on a beautiful mouth must begin with the subject of good oral hygiene. If beautiful lips part to reveal yellow, stained, or crooked teeth, then the whole effect is spoiled. Here are some suggestions to help maintain that beautiful smile.

1. See your dentist, preferably twice a year, for checkup and cleaning. He will also remove built-up tartar to safeguard you against gum disease. He will also instruct you in proper brushing and how to use dental floss. Dental floss helps keep down decay between the teeth and the resulting mouth odor from trapped food particles.

Ideally you should brush after every meal, but if it is inconvenient at lunch, then twice a day. Follow with a mouthwash for a really fresh feeling.

Smoking, in addition to being an obvious health hazard, yellows your teeth. An excess of coffee and tea will also stain your teeth. Use good judgment in cutting back or eliminating these caustic agents from your daily life.

If your teeth are crooked and need orthodontic attention, let me encourage you to get it at the earliest appropriate age. All too often, children develop inferiority complexes about their teeth which cut deeply into their self-image. They rarely smile for pictures and their whole personality can be affected.

Let me relate my own personal experience. I have always

had good straight teeth, but I used to have spaces between my upper front teeth which made me terribly self-conscious. Although the spaces were not that wide, to me they seemed like the width of the Grand Canyon. The spaces were particularly noticeable when I was photographed or appeared on TV. Every dentist that I consulted felt that the problem was so minor it was not worth the expense of braces and that my teeth were too good to ruin them with caps.

I was still not satisfied, but it was not until three years ago that my problem was solved. My dentist told me of a new process whereby the gaps could be filled in with a liquid substance which hardens and adheres to the sides of your own teeth. After having it done, I lost all self-consciousness about my teeth. It was amazing what that minute change did for me psychologically. Most of my friends never noticed the change until I pointed it out, but what a difference it made to me! My point is this: if you are self-conscious about any personal flaw, no matter how small, have it fixed. Your self-consciousness will vanish and your self-esteem will soar. (That's self-esteem, not vanity.)

The Lips

Remember—your lips are covered by the same delicate skin that covers your face; be sure and care for them also. Nothing is more unappealing than dry, cracked lips. Protection is the key word in maintaining beautiful, moist lips. Every night before retiring, apply a light coat of moisturizing cream to your lips to help keep them soft as you sleep. A clear lip gloss applied before your lip color will serve as protection during the day. Be especially careful to use protective creams during the winter and summer if you are active in outdoor activities and sports. Soft lips are essential for a beautifully made-up mouth.

Selecting Lip Color and Product

Years ago, women could select only one type of lip coloring—a lipstick in a tube—and the colors were limited. Today we could spend hours at a cosmetic counter choosing among hundreds of shades of lipsticks, glosses (stick, pot, or roll-on) and tubes of liquid color applied with its own applicator. The type of lip color you select is one of personal preference, but there are some general rules to follow.

Just as in fashion, lip color fads come and go. During the '30s and '40s the dark red mouth was in vogue, and how can we forget the deathly pale lips of the '60s? There will always be fads of one sort or another, and it is important to stay current by watching the fashion and beauty magazines.

The intensity and color you select should depend upon your hair and skin coloring. Dark-haired, olive-skinned women can wear the darker, more intense shades better than blondes with fair skin. The shade you select should flatter your skin tones and blend with your other makeup. Your lips should not stick out like a sore thumb, but beautifully complement the whole face. Your lip color should also be in the same color family as your blusher.

Applying Color and Shine

A lip brush or pencil is a must for a clean lip line. Invest in one or both and watch the definition of your mouth improve immediately. To use either one, hold it as you would a pencil and rest your little finger on your chin. If you have problems with your lip color running into the cracks around your mouth, then cover the edge of your lips with your foundation. Begin outlining your lips from the outer corner, progressing toward the center. Next fill in the center color. Placing a lighter shade in the bottom center lip gives a lovely highlight and adds a three-dimensional look. You can use your imagination and combine several shades for your best look. If you are to appear on stage, outlining your lips with a light brown pencil will give your mouth greater definition. This must be applied and blended carefully so as not to be very obvious.

Now that you have the color, finish it with the shine. Today's beautiful mouth looks moist and shiny. I recommend a lip gloss from a compact or pot for greater shine. If you prefer a less made-up look, just wear the gloss alone. I am never without gloss, even when I'm only at home doing my housework. It keeps your lips from drying out.

(Speaking of drying out, if you ride in parades or have to smile for a long time on stage, try rubbing a little vaseline on your gums. It will save you from some embarrassment, as it prevents your lips from drying in a smile on your gums!)

Lip Correction

If your mouth is less than perfect, here are a few ways to correct it. Again remember the principle of light and dark. The lighter shades will make your lips look larger; the darker shades, smaller. You may need to combine both to correct your problem.

Short thick lips	*Small upper lip*
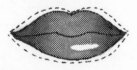	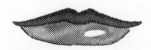
Cover lip line with same foundation used for face. Stop before middle of lips. Next apply color so that it gets darker and thinner toward the edge. *Do not* use color beyond natural lip line.	Line upper lip with a color of the same tone but two shades darker than regular lipstick. Using a brush and regular color, blend well to prevent outline from being obvious.
Heavy upper lip; drooping corners	*Thin lips; wide mouth*
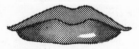	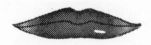
To balance the droop of upper lip add darker tone to lower-lip corners. Shape corner edges of bottom lip by lining it with a color the same tone, but two shades darker than regular shade. Stop before lip line turns downward. Blend and lighten color toward center of lips.	To correct for thin lips, follow procedure for small upper lip. Then outline lower lip. Stop short of corners. Fill in color and blend. To correct for wide mouth, place foundation on outside edges of mouth. Then using a brush to apply color, keep the tone darker in center and lighter toward corners.

Note: Reshape only those areas of lips that are noticeably irregular. Don't try to correct the shape of your entire mouth.

HANDS AND NAILS

I cannot leave this chapter without mentioning a related area of personal grooming—beautiful hands. Rough, red hands and broken, chipped nails can completely ruin all of your grooming efforts. It is important, therefore, to care for your hands and nails on a regular basis. I recommend a manicure once a week and prompt attention to broken, chipped nails or polish. It is a matter of personal preference whether you wear colored nail polish, but for the prettiest hands, try the look of clear polish at least.

Long, beautiful nails are a sign of femininity and are highly desirable, but don't get carried away and grow fangs! They are neither attractive nor functional. They are an impossibility when it comes to housework, typing, or just fastening a button. Keep your nails at a reasonable length and in proportion to your hands.

Nail color fads come and go. Keep abreast of the fashion, but wear what looks best with your skin tones. Please—no greens, blues, or other garish colors!

We all have problems with cracked, broken or splitting nails. First, to strengthen the nails, take protein supplement and gelatin tablets if necessary. If a nail cracks at the side, mend it by applying a coat of clear polish, then placing a small piece of tissue over the crack, molding it to the nail. After it dries, trim it and apply a second coat for strength. Nail-mending kits are available from several cosmetic companies.

Just a word about nail-biting. It is neither attractive nor healthy, and it generally reflects a person who is nervous or lacks confidence. If you have this problem, follow whatever course is necessary to break the habit. The total you will be so much more attractive.

PEDICURES

Feet may not be considered the most beautiful part of the body, but they do show from time to time and require proper attention. Give yourself a pedicure about once every two weeks. Soaking your feet in warm soapy water in preparation for the pedicure feels especially good and cleans the nails and softens the cuticles as well. Use a good brush for cleaning. Cut the toenails straight across to avoid ingrown nails. Remove calluses and thick dead skin with a pumice stone and follow with a lotion. Polish will add an extra touch of glamor to an otherwise unglamorous area.

Conclusion

It has been said that "beauty is only skin deep." I totally disagree. A woman's real beauty must come from within the inner you. But you cannot disregard the importance of the outer beauty that is you. Remember—you are a Designer creation, a one-of-a-kind original. Make the most of what God has given you; accept it and use it for His glory.

4

Hair Care and Styling

Gayelord Hauser, internationally acclaimed beauty and
health expert, believes there is no other single feature that
can do so much for a woman's looks as a mass of sweet-
smelling, shining hair. He maintains that there is no feminine feature that can glamorize, minimize or balance facial
shortcomings as can beautiful hair. He suggests that, in the
same way that a good frame can bring out and highlight a
picture, just so beautiful hair can frame and highlight a
woman's face and make an almost beautiful face into ex-
traordinary beauty.

Rubens, Renoir, Degas, and scores of other great artists
have dramatized women's hair in spectacular and dazzling
ways. Have you heard someone's hair described as being
titian-colored? This derives from the name of the artist
Titian who lived about 1477 through 1576, a Venetian
painter who gave his women subjects such fiery-colored
halos that his name has since become synonymous with
auburn, coppery-red hair.

Writers and poets have also focused on the hair of their
heroines—they delight in describing golden hair, flowing

Grateful acknowledgment is made to Gary Hottinger, Nine Hundred
West Salon, Austin, Texas, for his contribution to this chapter.

tresses, silken locks. Present-day artists and photographers play up the highlights in a woman's hair. And in the pages of history, certain eras have come to be identified by their characteristic hair styles. We think for instance of the Victorian Age and the women with their Gibson Girl pompadours; or the Southern belle with curls bouncing at the nape of her neck Scarlett-style as portrayed in *Gone With the Wind.* Puritan women wore prim buns; pioneer femininity expressed itself in sunbonnet and frizzed-out bangs. Mention shingled bobs and we immediately see flapper girls.

Certainly it is true that hair establishes an image for its wearer. With just a little experimenting on your own you can easily see how you can change your appearance by the way you wear your hair. You can make yourself appear severe and rather unapproachable, pretty and pleasing, exciting and fiery, chic and stylish. Very few things establish a woman's lifestyle and personality more than this mighty symbol of femininity.

What do we do then to attain the kind of hair, the shape and style hair that is easy to live with, that looks great at all times and requires a minimum amount of effort and care? Important questions.

We all know that it takes months to gain a perfect figure via diet and an exercise program. We know too that if we are born with a too prominent nose or some other facial defect we want to correct, weeks of hospitalization and major surgery can be required (should we be able to afford it—and it is very costly). Fortunately, hair is the one thing about ourselves that we can easily do something about through a visit to a reputable beauty salon and placing ourselves in the hands of a competent stylist. Even then, hair's best outer appearance, just as the figure's, comes from the inside and good care.

HAIR HEALTH

We begin with an understanding of hair health. A healthy head of hair will also be beautiful hair. It wouldn't make any difference if you had the most sought-after hair stylist in all the world and could afford to pamper yourself with the finest hair beauty products, if your hair wasn't healthy you would continue to have hair problems and not look your best. Oftentimes women are inclined to blame the weather or their hairsprays or shampoos if their hair looks dull and lifeless. The fault, in all likelihood, does not lie with those factors but rather with basic hair health.

I was fortunate to learn very early the importance of an inside approach to hair health and beauty and the contribution a well-balanced diet makes to the condition of my hair. Medical doctors acknowledge that vitamin and mineral deficiencies show up readily in an individual's hair. Certain hair tests can actually show what your body lacks. For example, you may be eating properly but your body not assimilating the minerals and vitamins in your food. Or your doctor may find an imbalance in your body's metabolism and give you the help you require.

My stylist informs me that hair is like a tape; it will register just what has happened and is happening to my body—what I am putting into it, what I am failing to give it, whether or not I am going through a very severe emotional shock or some degree of stress and trauma. You make a giant step in the right direction to real hair health and beauty when you recognize and understand this fact.

Other factors can contribute to hair problems, of course: sprays, tinting, bleaching, bad perms, teasing, drying, humidity, and so on. But most hair problems can be corrected and controlled by starting on the inside and checking one's diet. Replace empty starches and sugars and nutritionless foods with whole grains, fruits, juices, honey, vegetables, vegetable oils, and proteins. Always remember that your hair, like any other part of your body, is nourished by what goes into your body. A high protein diet or protein powder supplement will reward you with beautifully shining hair, as well as good skin and strong nails.

You really are what you eat. Everything that makes your hair grow, or go, is going to be determined by what happens to that hair follicle just beneath the scalp. In the regular, 1,000-day cycle of hair growth, you are constantly shedding old hair to make way for new hair. Health is a key factor, so if you are experiencing abnormal hair loss, check with your doctor and work to solve the underlying problem. Many women have experienced traumatic hair problems by going on crash diets and creating an imbalance in the body system through loss of essential proteins, vitamins and minerals. If you have recently come through an illness, a heart attack, major surgery, or even prolonged serious mental strain, you can also expect hair loss and other hair problems. Take heart, however, and realize that with adequate rest, a high protein diet, and the right medical or psychiatric care your body will soon respond and your hair will show improvement.

Proteins and Vitamins and Minerals

Did you know that your hair is about 97 percent protein? There is widespread general agreement that you should learn to think protein before you think anything else for hair health. One beauty expert recommends eating one-half gram of protein daily for every pound you weigh. Your body does not store protein, and your personal needs depend upon your height, weight, and body build. Meat, fish, fowl, milk, cheese, eggs, raw grains, nuts, seeds, and beans have traditionally been the best sources of protein. Wheat germ, I have learned recently, has a high quality protein value and stimulates hair growth.

Often we forget that our bodies require plenty of water—ideally, six glasses a day. If you have a problem with dry hair, lack of water could be the reason. That comes as a surprise to many women who have not made the connection between the two.

Healthy hair requires iron, and vegetable fats are also vitally important to shiny hair. Your hair actually craves fats; without them, you can be certain your hair is going to be dull, dry, listless and limp. Eat unsaturated fats; they are low in cholesterol but full of vitamin E, which I have discovered is good for every part of my body and also does wonders for my hair.

The value of lecithin is just beginning to be recognized. Lecithin helps to keep the fat moving off of us, but it's also marvelous for thickening up and shining the hair. It contains choline and inositol, two of the B-complex vitamins; and the B's are most essential to beautiful hair.

Hair experts will tell you that the B vitamins are basic to the best hair health. Some of the world's best-known hairdressers suggest B vitamins for their clients as part of their beautiful-hair program. While your particular hair color is inherited, the vitamins and minerals your body receives provide for the individual color-making factories located in each of your hair follicles. It has been proven that hair can turn from premature gray back to its natural color by the addition of the B vitamins in the form of supplements and the foods which supply ample quantities of such necessary vitamins and minerals. There are other anti-gray hair factors such as pantothenic acid, para-amino-benzoic acid, and folic acid (according to such nutrition experts as Gayelord Hauser and Adelle Davis and the writings of Linda Clark and Mary Ann Crenshaw).

I hope I have convinced you that right eating will do wonders for your hair, that it's the place to begin on a hair-improvement program as we work towards a better total you. Working from the inside out through more careful attention to what you eat won't bring instantaneous results, of course. But there are some things you can do while waiting for your new resolve and efforts toward hair health to take over.

CHOOSING THE RIGHT HAIRDRESSER

The choice of a good hairdresser, one in whom you have confidence, is extremely important and will do much for your overall outlook. But how do you find the right one? When in the market for a new hairdresser I usually look around and ask several women whose hair I admire where they have their hair done. I can't imagine any woman taking offense at being asked this question because it pays both her and the hairdresser a well-deserved compliment. That woman's hairdresser may not necessarily make an impression on you, but some careful looking around will usually be worth the effort if you do not already have a hairdresser in whom you have confidence.

After narrowing down the possibilities, I go in for a consultation, but I would not advise any drastic changes the first time he works on you. I believe it is wise for the hairdresser to get to know you a little—your lifestyle, the way you dress, speak, act, and the way you relate to your hair. The alert stylist will pick up on you from these clues and be better able to help you determine the way you wish to wear your hair and the way, therefore, that it should be cut and shaped.

Special Hair Problems

One of the first things necessary to help problem hair is for the hairdresser to analyze the condition of your hair and scalp. After this determination is made, he is in a better position to recommend that the dead dry ends be cut, and what beauty care products to use to help your hair from the outside, and what other procedures are necessary to bring your hair into better condition.

Oily hair, dry hair, a receding hairline, a widening part, hair that is going gray, cowlicks, hair breakage, overbleached hair, dandruff, too-thin hair—these and other hair problems will be helped by using hair products that have a pH balance of 4.5 to 5.5. In skin-care products as well as hair products, we should be aware of the importance of pH value—the measure for the chemical balance provided by nature for the protection of our skin and hair. The chemical symbol, pH, describes the relative acidity or alkalinity of your skin or of a product. How to keep the correct acidity is a problem your hairdresser is best qualified to deal with.

One of the reasons so many women encounter hair problems—split ends, dryness, hair breakage, and other undesirable conditions is that the pH balance has been disturbed. Many highly alkaline hair cosmetic products are readily available at the cosmetic counters and are damaging to the hair's natural acidity.

Fragile, overprocessed hair can be helped with correctly acid-balanced shampoos, protein and acid conditioners—actually any product with an acid pH.

Color-treated hair needs special care. It should be kept covered when you are in the sun. Remember also to keep your dryer set at warm; hot hair dryers are very hard on hair.

Oily hair requires especially careful watch over one's diet. An oily head of hair requires more frequent shampoos, every day if necessary. Nothing is more unattractive than dull oily hair. If you have oily hair you will also need to be careful to keep it off your face and shoulders or pimples and other similar skin problems are likely to occur.

Flaking and excessive dandruff really require medical treatment. Usually such problems are caused by an imbalance of hormones, improper diet, or nervous tension. If the problem is not severe, then one's hairdresser can help with the recommendation and use of the right hair care products.

Do not become impatient while waiting for the condition of your hair to improve. If you are concentrating on better nutrition, making certain you are getting the necessary vitamins and minerals, and receiving proper care, then you will see changes taking place. In some women this may take six months to a year, but the wait is worth it. Your hair didn't go bad overnight, and the condition will not change or improve overnight.

HAIRCUT AND STYLING

When you have found the right hairdresser and he or she has had time to get to know you, the two of you can decide about the cutting and shaping you want and need.

What you want and actually what you need may be two different things. Describe as closely as possible to your hairdresser what you have in mind. Communicate your feelings. Women have often been caught in the rut of conformity when it comes to changes in makeup and hair.

When a woman decides she needs to update or change the way she looks, more often than not she begins with the decision to do something about her hair. Years ago when a woman was depressed she went out and bought a new hat or dress. Today's woman is more likely to try a new hair style. My hairdresser tells me women come to him and say, "I want desperately to do something that is different. Just help me!"

A good stylist will look at the *Vogue* magazine his patron

is clutching and try to analyze both the woman sitting in his chair and the model she wants to copy. He might say to you, "This model has this type of hair and you have this type. . . . I'm not going to be able to give you that look, therefore—at least not exactly. But we'll get close to it." If, however, the look is all wrong for the woman in his chair, the wise hairdresser will take the time and make the effort to help his client realize what is best for her.

Actually the look in *Vogue* and other fashion magazines is the person. No amount of glamorizing by the most capable stylist is going to make a woman something that she cannot be if she is not that style, that type of person. It would be totally wrong. The recognition must come then that we must be totally ourselves and work within our limitations *and* our own unique possibilities. The hairdresser will work to bring out our best features and minimize whatever it is that makes us uncomfortable. It is up to you to tell him what that might be—your age, the type of hair you have (fine, coarse, thick, or thin), your bone structure, your height, your figure. All of these things must enter into a woman's choice of hair shape, cut and style.

The look most women seem to want today is one that says she has total hair freedom. She wants to know that if she gets out in the wind, she'll still have her style. She wants the kind of hair that men like to run their hands through, hair that moves and flows. In the many phases of hair styles that women have gone through, particularly in recent years, that total hair freedom look has not been possible. We really want to get away from "hairdressing" per se. Now that we've entered an era where this simple natural look for hair is back, the wise woman of today will work to keep it that way. It comes, however, with the right haircut.

Getting the cut you want depends not only on the hairdresser, but also on you. Educate yourself about your own head of hair. Does your hair wave easily or not? How does it react to weather—to moisture in the air or to dryness? Do you have some natural curl? Is your hair limp or lively after the first day of a new set? Do you require just a body permanent or more curl?

Your haircut must be suited to the texture and mass of your hair, to its condition, and the way it behaves. And, as has already been emphasized, the right cut should suit you —your face, the relationship to your whole body, your personality and lifestyle.

It is safe to say that the right haircut can do more for your hair than anything else. You need to feel comfortable with your hair style, and the right cut will achieve that. Perhaps you don't like your jawbone, or your nose, or having your ears exposed; the hairdresser will take all these things into consideration if you just share your feelings with him before he begins. The look you want as today's woman doesn't require fighting your hair or defying it; rather, work for change in a finished style that complements you and keeps you current with the trends. There should be involvement between you and your hairdresser so that no mistakes are made. The right cut will keep your new style in shape and leave your hair easy to set. It should also allow the style to fall naturally into place after brushing and should blend together without breaks.

According to my own stylist, in whom I have great confidence, there are really only two basic kinds of cuts. It can be cut into one length, or it can be cut into layers of different length.

Short layered hair needs to be cut every three to four weeks, depending on how fast your hair grows, in order not to grow out of the shape that was cut into it. It is recommended that hair be cut while wet and that the ends be blunted (that is, that the exact style be cut into the ends of the hair whether layered or one length). Razors are *not* recommended for cutting, as they damage the hair. Small scissors are to be preferred, with the stylist cutting little sections of the hair at a time. The short scissors give a greater degree of control.

Let's Brush up on Brushing

One hundred strokes a day! Right or wrong? Grandmother would tell you that the young women of her day just knew that brushing those one hundred strokes a day was the thing that made their hair so beautiful. There are differences of opinion. Brushing is, of course, just one more way to keep hair shiny, to lessen the dangers of tangles, and

to aid circulation. Brushing does draw natural oils from our
scalp and distribute them along the hair shaft. This can be
a blessing to the woman who suffers from dry hair problems; but it would make the oily hair on another woman become more oily. Most hairdressers today will tell you that
the one hundred strokes a day is a thing of the past; but
what they will recommend instead is gentle brushing, twice
a day, perhaps a few dozen strokes.

The long-haired woman would benefit from bending at
the waist, letting her hair fall forward, and brushing from
back to front. Those of us who wear our hair shorter could
do the same. The increased blood circulation certainly benefits the scalp, but the important thing is not to neglect gentle
brushing with the right kind of brush.

What is the right kind of brush? Beauty experts are in
general agreement on two basic types: the natural bristle
brush with smooth rounded ends which certainly cannot
harm hair and the plastic-bristle brushes with rubber bases
and wide-apart plastic prongs that go through the hair
easily and prevent tangling. Never brush wet hair. And do
not use natural boar bristle brushes on wet hair—only dry.
Use the comb, working carefully if there are any tangles,
and work from the bottom upward bit by bit.

What About Heated Rollers, Blow Dryers, and Curling Irons?

Electric rollers and curling irons have become essential
tools for many women today. A word of caution is in order.
Use of these devices can result in severe damage to the hair
should the rollers or iron be too hot for the hair shaft. Look
for electric rollers that have a wax substance on the inside of
the rollers which indicate when the roller is at the right
temperature to use. Such rollers are very mild in compari-
son.

Temperature-controlled curling irons are to be preferred
for home use. The barrel of the iron should be smooth, but
stay away from those with Teflon coating; if your hair is
even slightly dirty, or the Teflon gets dirty, it will be melted
into the hair cuticle. If the curling iron is used properly and

the temperature control set so that it is not too hot, the possibility of damage to the hair is lessened. My hairdresser advises against using curling irons on long hair. Curling irons are fine for short hair provided you know how to work with it—it takes practice but can be a lifesaver for the woman with a busy schedule.

Learning to use a blow dryer is a skill most women can develop. Many of the pretty, natural-looking hairstyles you see today are achieved with heated rollers, curling irons and blow dryers. But remember, caution is the watchword. You have already learned that excessive heat can severely dry one's hair. Use pH-balanced, approved hair care products and always be careful when doing any home heat styling.

Body Waves and Permanent Waves

A body wave means control, in varying degrees depending on how long the perm is left in. A body wave and a permanent wave differ only in the size of the rod on which the hair is wound. For hair with lots of curl, the hairdresser will use a small rod. Hair with moderate curl requires larger rods. For a body wave only, even larger rods are used, and the permanent must be processed to the perfect time.

A little explanation about the chemical content of hair may help the reader to understand what a body wave or longer-lasting permanent wave does. Earlier I told you that the hair is about 97 percent protein. These protein molecules are held together by chemical links which are the building blocks of the hair shaft, and the way in which these chemical links position the protein molecules determines the straightness or curliness of our hair. Body waves and permanent waves rearrange these protein molecules and the bonds connecting them. The solutions applied in various stages of the procedure, the size of the rods used, and the careful timing all have their part in doing for your hair what nature may have failed to do to enable you to wear your hair the way you want it.

When carefully done and properly conditioned, body waves and permanents can do much to enhance a woman's appearance and add to ease in the care and handling of her hair. They can give body to limp hair, make thin hair seem thicker, and form waves and curls in straight hair.

Remember That You Cannot Hurry Beauty

When I look at the Miss America photographs of my reigning year and then at my image in the mirror today, I see the same Donna, but different somehow. I know that there are several reasons for this—there has been a maturing and a learning process. My hairdresser describes it as more determination now, more "polish" and more freshness. I ask myself how can that be? I was so determined then, and I was certainly young and what would be called fresh and possessing a youthful bloom.

I did wear my hair differently then. I note the difference that makes. We women are conscious of trends for the time in which we live; we are a style-conscious breed, and hair is part of our social and cultural statement. Yes, definitely, and it changes with time.

We have seen the totally sculptured, coiffured look replaced by a style more adaptable to a woman's lifestyle. Yet it enables her to look fantastic, and it is one that can be achieved in a relatively small amount of time and maintained with ease. This is, I believe, for the good. The average woman wants to be able to control her hair so that she doesn't have to rely upon a hairdresser everytime she goes someplace. Women want hair that looks like hair instead of a plastered halo. We want to live enjoyable lives and not be held back by our hair style.

In Summary

You are unique, and so is your hair. You must be the ultimate judge of what you are going to do with your head of hair. But on the basis of conversations I've had with women through the years, the tremendous amount of research, time and money spent to develop hair care products, and the vast number of books and magazine articles one can read on the subject of hair I am led to believe that looking good and feeling good starts at the top. When you know that your hair is healthy and looks pretty, then you feel good about yourself.

In 1976 eleven hairdressers met together with bartenders and taxi drivers in San Diego, California. They had been selected to participate in a pilot program conducted by a family counseling center. It seems that people in these three occupations—diverse as they may be—hear a continuing series of personal problems day after day. They are, in many ways and to some extent, amateur psychologists and counselors.

The group learned that basic human needs are love, security, significance and rest. They discovered too that emotions can quickly become overwhelming when an individual is threatened.

The point of my calling this to your attention is simply that when you know you look your best, you are going to be in a better position to meet the demands of life. A trip to the hairdresser may be just the psychological boost you need to help you become totally you, with all that that represents mentally, physically, and spiritually.

In the practical aspects of living, we cannot afford to deceive ourselves. To want to look our best is a sign of good mental health. The tone of our life is set not so much by external circumstances as it is by the attitude we have toward ourselves. For good reason the Bible says that as a man thinketh in his heart, so is he (Prov. 23:7). Think poorly of yourself and your attitude toward others will be affected accordingly. The opposite of that, of course, is to think well of yourself, to have that self-love which Dr. Robert Schuller of the famed Garden Grove Community Church calls the dynamic force of success.

Such a proper self-love could begin for you at the point of having a better self-image.

p.s. Every woman should learn to care for her hair on a daily basis and not be totally dependent upon her hairdresser except for cuts, perms, color, etc. Be in control of your hair and you are in control of your time.

5

Wardrobe Coordination

"Fashion is really how you wear clothes; everything is up to you. Don't let your clothes wear you. You must learn to relate fashion to yourself in the simplest, most comfortable, most attractive terms. Don't let fashion frazzle you. It should be easy. Easy and comfortable. The key is 'Simple is best; less becomes more.'"

These are the words of Halston, and he is right: simplicity is the essence of elegance. And if anyone should know, it's Halston, hailed as America's preeminent fashion designer and a member of the Coty Award Hall of Fame, the highest honor bestowed upon a designer.

Although we cannot all afford to buy designer originals, we can study the lines, colors, and fabrics used by the designers and make them guidelines for our own wardrobe coordination. Also by studying the designers, we can stay abreast of the latest solid fashion trends with an eye to keeping our wardrobes updated. This is important whether we buy or make our own clothes.

CLOTHING—YOUR PERSONAL STATEMENT

In an earlier chapter we discussed how important a part good carriage plays in nonverbally communicating confidence and self-esteem. Equally as important is good grooming and attractively coordinated clothing. In fact, clothing style and appearance are usually an accurate statement of (1) personality, (2) self-esteem, (3) personal background and convictions, (4) lifestyle, and (5) social class. There are exceptions to every rule, of course.

Psychologically speaking, the right clothing can make the difference between a positive, self-confident you or a depressed, self-conscious you. When you know you look great, the psychological boost will help put you at your best for that important date, interview or social affair. There have been days when I have gone back home on my lunch hour and changed because I've not felt good about the way I've looked.

THE TOTAL PICTURE

When selecting clothing, I feel that it is important to remember Halston's rule—you wear the clothing, don't let it wear you. You have succeeded in putting together a total look in clothing, accessories, hair and makeup when the first impression is "Wow—you look fantastic" instead of "Oh, I like your dress." Each element is an intricate part of the total picture. For these reasons, I prefer simple line, good fabric, and tasteful use of color. I avoid loud brassy colors and extremely bold prints as I feel that they will overpower and detract from the overall effect.

CLOTHING—THE BLUE CHIP INVESTMENT

It is fairly realistic to estimate that you will spend one-fourth to one-third of your yearly income on clothing, depending upon your job and social activities. In view of the cost of today's fashions, it is an important investment. Halston says: "Quality clothes will reward you, not only by looking exquisitely beautiful but by lasting longer. Inexpensive clothes usually perform badly because of poor fabric and construction. If you have only a limited amount of money to spend on clothing, I would suggest you buy a designer pattern and some good fabric and sew yourself a smashing outfit." Let me urge you then to develop a "blue chip" philosophy when making clothing decisions. 1. Be very selective according to style, fit, and color for your face and figure. 2. Buy quality, classic garments that will give you years of good wear (even if you have to have fewer in number) and that will coordinate with your existing wardrobe. 3. Avoid fashion fads that will be out of style in one year. 4. Absolutely love every wardrobe item before purchase; otherwise it will stay in the closet and you will suffer a financial investment loss. These theories apply also if you make your own clothes—a valuable asset. I would encourage all women to learn some basic sewing skills at least; you can cut down on costly alteration, mend your own clothes, and have a better concept of good clothing construction.

TAKING STOCK

To plan and coordinate a good wardrobe you must begin by taking an inventory of what you have to work with and what needs to be eliminated. I try to do my inventory just prior to the buying period of each season. The fact that it is difficult to remember from year to year what we have in our wardrobe can lead to unnecessary duplication and unwise buying. Make an inventory check list in advance so that you will know what items you need to purchase or replace and can plan your budget ahead. You will avoid costly finance charges when paying out an account. Also, learn to extend your wardrobe with separates and coordinates. Study what you have; then decide what items can be purchased that will offer freshness and versatility. New accessories such as shoes, scarfs, flowers, belts, and jewelry will add a fresh look. Don't forget to inventory your lingerie and sleepwear from time to time also.

KEEP IT STRAIGHT

Now that you have completed your wardrobe inventory and assessed your needs, why not arrange your closet and drawers so as to save you time?

I have found these categories work best for me:

1. Seasonal storage (in closet with clothes cleaned before storage and protected from dust by bags).

2. Clothing in use, arranged according to type, i.e., Sunday dresses, daytime dresses, pantsuits, co-ordinates, pants, blouses, robes.

3. Coats and evening wear, in a different closet, or if that

is not possible for you, in the least used (perhaps the most inaccessible) part of your closet.

One little hint: keep plastic dry cleaning bags over clothes to help prevent wrinkling and accumulation of dust, particularly on those items worn less frequently and on seasonal clothes. Caution: plastic bags are not to be used over furs; wrap them in cloth so that the fur can breathe or put them in storage.

From time to time you will have to put things back in order. Don't wait too long. You *can* avoid those endless searches for that lost skirt or blouse. When you are on a busy schedule, fewer frustrations help!

I make it a practice to check once a week for clothing that needs washing, dry cleaning, mending, or ironing. This has saved many moments when I am in the process of getting ready and on a time schedule. A hand-held steamer is a must for traveling and fast touchups. And while I'm mentioning clothing, don't forget your shoes—an important part of your total picture. How often a person's appearance is spoiled by scuffed shoes and heels that are run down. Don't neglect this aspect of good grooming.

RECYCLE YOUR WARDROBE DOLLARS

In recent years the term recycling has come into prominence. We recycle aluminum, glass, and paper—why not clothing? As you look over your wardrobe you will no doubt come across many items that you no longer wear for one reason or another. If you are not going to use something, recycle it—there are so many people who are in need of clothing. Why not share for profit or as a tax-deductible contribution? Here are some of the ways I make my wardrobe dollars go further—it's just good sense. And if you haven't worn a garment in over a year or two, chances are that it will continue to catch dust.

1. Donations to Goodwill, Salvation Army, or some other reputable organization. Your own church may have a place where clothing is collected for needy individuals. Perhaps you know someone who wears your size who would welcome the items you no longer wish to keep. The point is, they are serving no useful purpose in your closet or drawers, so re-

cycle them. If you give these items to a charitable organization, they are prepared to give you a tax receipt.

2. Next-to-new type consignment. Many of my friends
and acquaintances have great success in doing this. These
are legitimate business operations which require that the
clothes be in style, freshly laundered and pressed, and/or
dry cleaned, and in salable condition. They, in turn, help
you determine the sale price, place the items on their racks,
and give you back a nice percentage after the items have
sold. It is great fun to receive that check; not only have you
gotten wear from the clothes but also a small dollar return
on your clothing investment.

Some of these places also accept handbags, jewelry, belts
and other accessories. While you are delivering your items,
keep your eyes open—you may find a treasure yourself.
There are women just like yourself who made unwise purchases in the past, or have found they no longer can fit into a
certain item, or have lost interest in it. Such stores, for the
most part, are quite selective in what they take. You might
surprise yourself and save some money.

3. Garage sales. These have skyrocketed in popularity,
now that many families have discovered they are not only
fun but profitable! By going in with someone you expand
your variety and share the work. It's not unusual to make
several hundred dollars from a well-organized, advertised
sale.

Back to the Basics

With your inventory completed and unusable items dis-
carded, you should have a clear idea of what you have to
build on.

A good, versatile wardrobe will have as its foundation
several items in your basic color—brown, black or gray, as
determined by what is best with your hair and skin coloring.
White is also an important color for a few separates as it offers endless variety with any color.

Now determine your complementary colors—the colors
that accent your eyes or set off your skin and hair. I have
found that vivid clear colors around my face are great—
even a blouse or scarf gives a refreshing lift. Stay away from

colors that are too harsh for your coloring or wash out your skin tones. (For girls entering pageants, vivid colors are better for stage in talent and swimsuit competitions. Save the lighter pastels for evening gown competition, and avoid black as a competition gown.)

Florals and prints are nice but very limiting unless they are separates and can be combined with solid-colored items.

"Thank you—I'm just looking" is a phrase that we commonly use when shopping. It can be positive or negative— let me explain. It is positive when you have a good idea of what items, styles, and colors you are looking for to expand your wardrobe. It's best not to shop in haste but take plenty of time. Visit a number of stores and compare styles and prices before making a purchase. Look until you are absolutely satisfied with your selections. Anything less may lead to a costly mistake.

"I'm just looking" can be a dangerous statement if you are a "clothesaholic," a woman who has little control over her desire for new clothes. Many use it as a psychological boost for depression. Some people eat; others buy clothes. But momentary delight soon changes to gloom when the bills start rolling in. To help you keep track of your clothing purchases, jot them down in a book each month listing price and date of purchase. It's a realistic approach to keeping your spending under control. Of course, paying cash only will help keep you from getting in over your head in bills and finance charges.

WHAT ABOUT BARGAINS AND SALES?

At certain times of the year—January, July and August— you will be able to pick up what I call real bargains. This is a particularly good time to pick up a great designer dress that may have been out of your price range at its regular price. You would not, however, be getting a bargain if your purchase was a fashion fad good for only one season. Staying with classic lines and styles is always safe. Remember that tastes and trends may change from season to season and from year to year, but the basic rules do not.

Keep the following rules in mind regarding sale purchases. Avoid them *if:*

1. The item needs a major alteration job. The money saved on the item would then be consumed in the alteration costs. That is well and good *if* you really like the item and if you need it and *if* it looks right on you. Three big "ifs."

2. You wouldn't have bought it at its regular price! Either it looks really great on you and you are "sold" on it for what it is, not because it's on sale; or you *don't need* it.

3. You have to make major accessory purchases that will require an additional outlay of money you weren't figuring on spending, and the accessories may not go with other items in your wardrobe. A bargain ceases to be a bargain when we really don't need it, and when the cost incurred is no saving because we incur additional costs along the way (accessorizing, alterations, etc.).

ACCESSORIES: THE FINISHING TOUCH

You should take as much care in coordinating your accessories as you do with your clothing. These can make or break the total look. They add just the right sparkle, color, or contrast—the perfect finish for a great outfit.

Color

Color in accessories can be used to blend with your garments, or to contrast or pick up a certain color in a print or plaid. There are no hard and fast rules in fashion today governing this area; just use your best fashion taste and ask for assistance from your store fashion coordinator. It's always helpful to study fashion magazines and observe how the pros do it. One final hint—accessories should accent, not dominate the overall picture.

Scale

Always keep your accessories, especially handbags, in proportion to your size. Nothing looks sillier than to see a woman of five-foot height carrying a huge handbag that hangs down to her ankles. The opposite holds true for a larger woman: avoid the petite one.

Scarves, jewelry, flowers, bags—keep everything in proportion to your size.

Appropriateness

In addition to color and scale, appropriateness to the outfit and the occasion is essential. Casual fabrics and leather looks should not be mixed with elegant clothing. The reverse is true also.

Jewelry and Other Accessories

When it comes to jewelry, I caution women to buy with care. There is no reason you shouldn't start collecting a few really choice pieces of jewelry. This doesn't mean they have to cost a fortune, since even in costume jewelry of department store quality you can buy some really excellent pieces that will last a lifetime if given good care. Good jewels, jewelry store quality, will represent an investment that you can cherish and enjoy and pass on to your children and grandchildren. Jewelry gives a precise air, like a punctuation mark at the end of a sentence to emphasize a statement. You'll want to be more careful in future purchases of jewelry, always keeping in mind that quality is superimportant.

Sunglasses, fashion glasses, and hats would be considered as accessories also. If you wear glasses be sure that the frames are wide enough for your face and are an attractive color and shape for your face.

There is one general rule about accessories that you should know and follow: keep all accessories in proportion to your figure. Large woman—large accessories; medium woman—medium accessories; small woman—small accessories. That's not hard to remember, is it? Make accessories work for you, doing for you what needs to be done. And always keep your accessories as casual or as elegant as the occasion requires. Rhinestones and glitter after five only, please. Remember, too, that accessories can do wonders for less expensive clothes. Accessories are like the frosting on cake—hmmmm, great!

In accessorizing it's accent you are after, not clutter. Don't overdo it and try to wear all your jewelry at once. Be selective. Accessories should be fun—and interchangeable. They are a touch of polish and can make or break the total effect.

The Honest Art of Deception—Figure Camouflage!

I hope that, even while you're reading this book, you have launched yourself into a diet and exercise improvement program, but in the interim you can still look good with some skillful camouflage. Here are some general guidelines to follow:

1. *Evaluate your figure.* Study your figure; take inventory of its good points as well as those where it departs from perfection. You'll need tape measure, yardstick, bathroom scales, and a full-length three-way mirror. Be honest with yourself.
2. *Use line and color to de-emphasize figure imperfections.* Avoid repeating in your clothing a line you do not want noticed. For example, if you have a squared chin line, don't choose a square neckline. On the other hand, line and color can be used to create the impression of a perfectly proportioned figure. Some women may need to use broadening lines in the bust area and avoid such lines in the hip area to achieve the look of a more balanced figure. Apply the same principle to other figure problems.
3. *Wear clothing that fits properly.* A poor fit can destroy the entire impression you are working to create. Be sure you can move and sit comfortably in your clothes. Sleeves, collars, and waistline should fit smoothly without binding; set-in sleeves should hit the tip of your shoulder bone. Don't rely on manufacturer's sizes; their lines vary considerably. Buy only what fits *you.*

Always Consider the Fit

Please don't try squeezing into a size 10 when a 12 would be so much better. And don't talk yourself into going one size smaller on the rationale that you're going to lose. I'm glad you know you are going to lose, but delay your buying until such time as you actually do. Who knows? You might drop two or even three sizes!

Anything that is too tight, too loose, too short, or too long is going to distract from your total look and also your comfort. Pay attention to the way your clothes fit. When you are able to move about and breathe with ease, you'll stand, sit and move gracefully and reflect the knowledge that you have fashion self-confidence.

Body measurements have a sneaky way of changing. Be aware of this fact and keep that tape measure handy. Yes, it's ego-deflating to have to admit that you've jumped into another size or that your waistline has increased several inches. But the well-groomed, fluid look is what you are after, and it comes only through proper fit.

Line and Color

Two of the most important elements of camouflage are line and color.

Horizontal lines cut the figure, thus giving a shorter, wider effect as seen in this illustration.

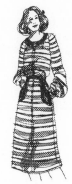

Horizontal lines give better proportion to too tall, too thin figure

Wear if: you are tall and slender and want to appear shorter and wider. Avoid vertical lines.

Avoid if: you are short and overweight—the optical illusion will cause you to look even shorter and wider. Wear vertical lines.

Remember these basic rules of color when selecting your wardrobe: Light colors advance and make things appear larger. Dark colors recede and make things appear smaller.

If tall and thin: wear lighter colors, mixing shades which will also break the vertical line. Avoid all black, navy or other colors of deep intensity in an overall outfit.

If short and stout: use the darker colors; avoid white and high-intensity lighter colors.

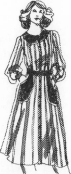

Vertical lines give flattering look to too heavy, too short figure

Prints and Fabrics

One word of warning about prints and stripes: please keep them in proportion to your size.

Larger women should stay away from heavy, thick fabrics as they add bulk. Stretch-knit pants and shiny materials are also a no-no as they will only accent your problems.

HEM LENGTH

Wear your hems in accordance with the fashion trends of the day, but adjust them to your individual height requirements. The taller woman usually looks good in all the new lengths. The medium to short woman would be well advised to wear her hems in proportion to her height, but within the general fashion trend range. Please don't date yourself by wearing short mini skirts when the trend is mid-calf. Regardless of the designer or manufacturing styles, hem lengths will generally be a universally agreed factor.

TRAVEL TIPS FOR THE WARDROBE

During my Miss America reign, I traveled some 250,000 miles. I learned very quickly the value of efficient packing. Here are some suggestions that will make your traveling easier.

1. Purchase sturdy, large wardrobe cases with strong fasteners and locks. They must be able to withstand weight and rough treatment.

2. Separate, if possible in different bags: (1) clothing, (2) accessories, blow dryers and other items of weight, and (3) cosmetics, which should be carried in a hand-held bag to prevent spilling (I usually carry this bag with me on the plane in case my luggage is lost).

3. Pack each garment on a hanger and cover with a plastic cleaning bag. This helps prevent wrinkles and makes unpacking at your destination a breeze.

4. Travel with steam iron, needle and thread, and any other emergency mending supplies you may need.

5. Coordinate your wardrobe in such a way as to elimi-

nate as many different pairs of shoes and purses as possible.

6. Travel with fabrics that don't wrinkle easily. Some that can be hand-washed are great.

7. Don't take too many clothes, but be prepared for every occasion.

SUMMARY

In conclusion, know your figure problems and learn how to work with them effectively. Keep up with fashion trends and always remember that the clothing you select and the manner in which you put yourself together are your personality statement. Be a careful buyer and recycle those wardrobe dollars.

As a child Donna was always underweight.

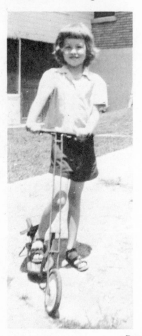

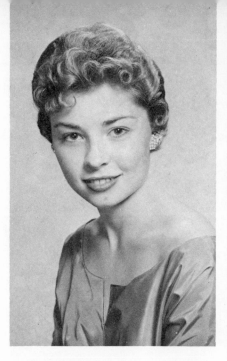

High school senior.

Donna won her first title at age 16—Miss Union County, El Dorado, Arkansas 1958.

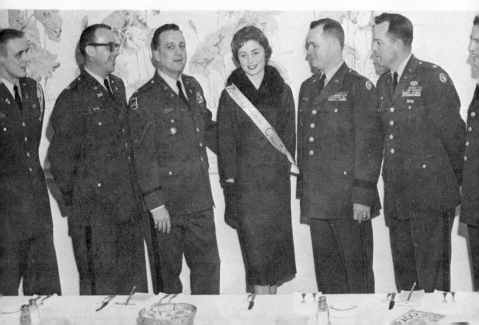

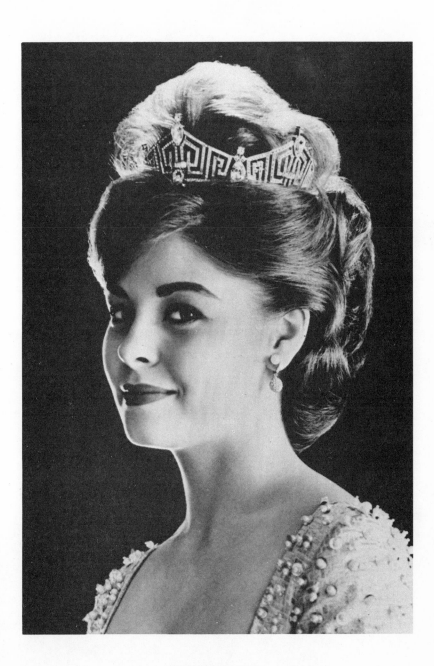

Miss America 1964

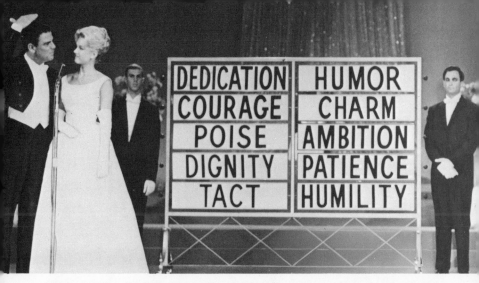

DEDICATION | HUMOR
COURAGE | CHARM
POISE | AMBITION
DIGNITY | PATIENCE
TACT | HUMILITY

As one of five finalists, Donna (far right) waits for her turn to speak on attributes a Miss America should possess. Each contestant had to choose one topic from the board; Donna's choice was "humility." Other finalists, from left, are Miss Arizona, Miss Tennessee, Miss Hawaii, and Miss District of Columbia.

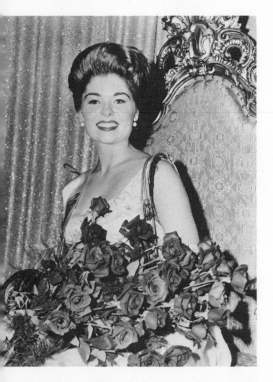

Miss America, seated on her official throne.

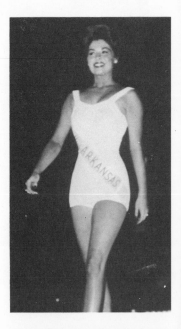

Preliminary swimsuit winner in Miss Arkansas and Miss America Pageants.

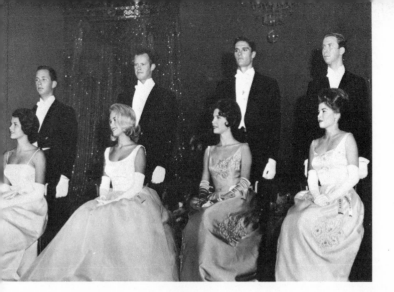

With parents, Hurley B. and Idelle Axum, at American
Bankers Convention in Washington, D.C., 1964.

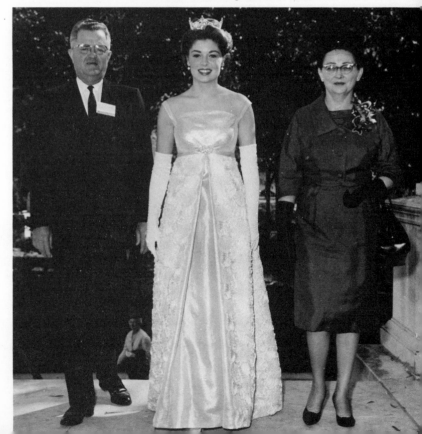

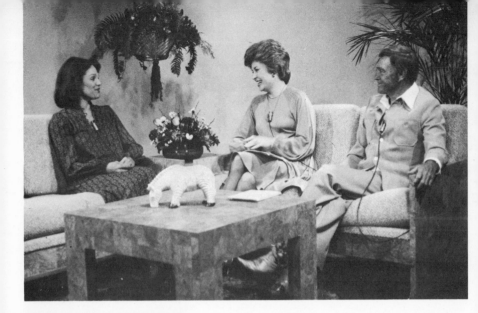

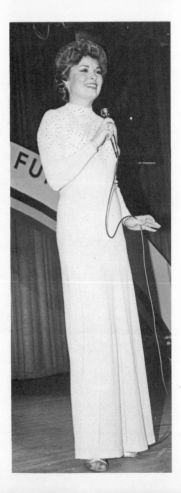

Above: Spring 1977 – Co-hostess and producer Donna Axum of "Noon" (KTBC-TV, Austin, Texas) with co-host Cactus Pryor and guest Valerie Harper "Rhoda." Left: August 6, 1977 – Donna serves as Austin Aqua Festival Beauty Pageant Vice-Commodore, emcee and singer (Photo by Joyce Marie Smith). Below: Donna with children, Gus Hurley and Lisa.

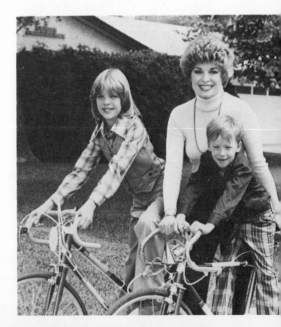

The Inner You

⌒ 6 ⌒

Beauty of Mind and Spirit

As a teenager I was walking along the beach in Florida one night enjoying the pounding of the surf. I looked up and there seemed to be eighteen billion stars up in the heavens. I recall now how small I felt then. My feet kicked up the sand as I hurried along. And then I was struck with the realization that there are multiplied thousands upon thousands of grains of sand along the beaches and seashores all over this vast universe. Stars and sand. Sand and stars. And people.

I stopped and just stood silently gazing upward for a few moments. I remember thinking finally: "God, You've created all this; and You've created me. You are infinite; and I am so finite. God, why did You create me? What is my purpose here on earth?"

Later, I stumbled across a psalm which expressed the same sort of thoughts: "O Lord our Lord, how excellent is thy name in all the earth! who hast set thy glory above the heavens. . . . When I consider thy heavens, the work of thy fingers, the moon and the stars, which thou hast ordained; What is man, that thou art mindful of him?" (Ps. 8:1, 3, 4a). The writer of that psalm was overcome with awe when he realized how tiny a part of this magnificent universe he was. That's just how I felt.

Question Time

I started asking myself some questions, and I remembered some words that hadn't made sense when I first read them. The writer had said something about being patient toward all that was unsolved in your heart. She had suggested that we learn to love the questions themselves and not seek to know *all* the answers. It was encouraging to realize that the point was to live the questions *now*. In the very living we would find the answers to our questions.

I have always been a seeking person. During my Miss America reign, my mother was questioned about my childhood and teenage years. Among other things, she told interviewers that I was born with something that keeps me going. One newspaper reporter said that, instead of waiting for something to happen, I climbed upon my own ladders of talent and determination until I was tall enough to poke my head into the crown!

Humility

I can still remember how thrilled I was as I sat on that huge stage in Convention Hall in Atlantic City as one of the five finalists in the 1963 Miss America Pageant. Thrilled, and excited, but somehow filled with an inner calm as I waited for Bert Parks to call my name for the final test. In those days questions were asked of the five finalists to determine speaking ability, poise, and intelligence before an audience. That year the usual question format was replaced with a word board instead. The board was rolled out on stage and positioned so that we were unable to see the words until we were at the mike with Bert. The board contained words depicting areas of character, such as *dignity, ambition, courage,* and *patience*. There were ten words in all. We were to select a word and tell what that word meant to us.

"Miss Arkansas," Bert called me to the mike. We chatted for a few moments, and then he asked me to turn and choose my word. My eyes quickly scanned the board of words remaining and came to rest on the one I knew I would select—*humility*. I chose the word because it reminded me of a dear friend in Arkansas named Phyllis Owen—"Chee Chee" as we called her. She was the very embodiment of the term. Here is the essence of what I said.

"We all have certain goals set for our lives, and we are all seeking to be successful in our respective fields. In order to do so we should all strive to be humble, for humility is the key to success in life. It's a desirable characteristic for people of all ages. And humility, though very, very obvious to others, is invisible to those who possess it."

Ironically, Phyllis was married that same night back in Arkansas, and she rushed back to a TV set in time to see me crowned. (She had asked me to sing for her wedding before I became Miss Arkansas.)

A spirit of humility is certainly a desirable quality for all women—unassuming, with awareness and consideration for people in all walks of life. By exercising a humble spirit we are always able to put ourselves in the other fellow's shoes and to see the world from his side of the street.

DETERMINATION

Determination? Yes, I do know what that is. I know of no successful individual, past or present, who has reached specific goals without applying heaping measures of self-discipline and a strong determination of will. During that three-year period when I was working toward the Miss Arkansas, Miss America goal, I kept this verse taped to my mirror and read it every day: "Keep everlastingly at it, allow nothing to discourage or deter you. Live it, sleep it, dream it—keep on and on and that goal will be yours" (author unknown).

TALENT

Talent? I am firmly convinced that God places within each of us certain unique abilities. Both the Apostle Paul and Peter emphasize this. Paul speaks of the assurance that God has given each of us the ability to do certain things well. Peter said almost the same thing: "God has given each of you some special abilities; be sure to use them to help each other, passing on to others God's many kinds of blessings" (1 Pet. 4:10, TLB).

I sang and danced my way through childhood. I loved entertaining people. Natural talents, gifts from the Creator —but I had to apply myself and work to develop and improve them. Leonardo da Vinci said, "Thou givest us everything at the price of an effort." I'll endorse that!

FAITH

In 1964, after I was named Miss America, life seemed to be filled with a storybook quality: events seemed to promise that glamor, beauty, success, and happiness would be mine forever after. Happiness forever after? Not necessarily so. Whether I liked it or not, being named Miss America changed my life forever. On that starry-eyed night of September 7, 1963, I did not have an inkling of the experiences that would unfold for me, during the next ten years in particular. I had known the heights of glamor and success, but I was also to experience the depths of failure. But through it all, there was one thing that sustained me. The poet calls it having a "heart full of faith within." I know now I could not have endured had it not been for my own personal faith in a God who does all things well.

Through the years, many women have admired the huge trophy and the beautiful Miss America crown in my home. We humans tend to put much emphasis on material things, frequently in excess. But I know the truth is that when we are stripped of our material possessions—as we all will be someday—it's not what we have nor what we've accomplished that is important, but what we are on the inside. The inner you is what really matters. It's not the clothing we put on our bodies, nor the ornaments with which we adorn ourselves, or the transportation that takes us down the street—it's how we relate to God and to our fellow man and how we respond to His will.

My own strong faith goes back to my childhood and upbringing. I am extremely thankful to my parents for the training they gave my sister and me. I appreciate their dili-

gence in setting the example of regular attendance in our
local Baptist church and in seeing that we learned the importance of the Bible as God's Word. My heart aches for
children and young people who are not given this kind of
foundation. The way to meet the crises events of life—and
everyone encounters them in different ways—is to begin
early to prepare for them. In my college years especially, I
learned the importance of the foundation my parents had
helped me build.

Certainly we do not grow in faith and develop our convictions merely through the religious heritage our parents
give us. But we are remiss as parents when we do not afford
our children the opportunity to learn about God and biblical
truths, to prepare for the challenges and reverses in life by
fortifying the inner person. By this means we develop character, acquire the ability to think clearly and with vital fore-
sight, build courage, determination and other virtues
essential to real beauty of mind and spirit.

To do anything vital in life, we must first obtain self-
mastery. It is essential to build up inner reserves. So many
of our failures result from impatience, or from hurried or
unwise decisions and from avoiding problems rather than
attacking them. Without a firm foundation of faith in an
all-knowing God, we can sink in trouble and end in ruin.

The relationships within our homes are tremendously important, for it is here we learn about the caring qualities of
love and of people helping one another. Here, too, we experience the importance of honesty and the fact that the
tapestry of life is made up of many hues—both bright events
and darker moments. And here can be instilled within us
that composure of mind and spirit that radiates peace when
we trust in the One who made us. I like what Peter said:
"Trust yourself to the God who made you, for he will never
fail you" (1 Pet. 4:19b, TLB).

WHAT REALLY IS BEAUTY?

The first half of this book concerned itself with our outward appearance, for good reason, but now we turn our
attention to inner beauty—the inner you.

Inner beauty is an elusive quality that needs to be developed. The kind of inner beauty I am talking about, and that Peter referred to, is the glow that radiates from the woman who has entrusted her life into Christ's hands—the inner *peace* that she feels because she knows that God is with her, giving her life *joy*. This kind of beauty is irresistible. Whether she is physically endowed or not, such a woman has an indescribable quality about her that sets her apart.

I have a friend who says God wants to make the best of us, but we have to be willing to give him the worst of us. The Apostle Paul says that we are to be "tools in the hands of God, to be used for his good purposes" (Rom. 6:13, TLB). In other words, God is the transforming business, and his method is to begin with an inward transformation that manifests itself in outward ways. The point of beginning is self-acceptance. That's one of the reasons I believe it is so important for women to learn a few things about themselves so that they can like themselves. God made us just the way we are for good reason—that's the way He wants us.

SELF-CONFIDENCE

There are specific things you can do to develop beauty of mind and spirit. First of all, you can recognize your worth to God. You may have failed Him in some ways in the past, but that doesn't need to characterize the present and the future. Don't carry an unnecessary burden of guilt for real or imagined past sins or failures. Inner healing, about which so much is now being said and written, can begin now.

Another important way to improve your feelings and attitude about yourself is to recognize the unique gifts God has entrusted to you. He put them into your makeup; now it's up to you to cultivate them. Many resources are within your reach to help you develop your creative talents, hobbies and skills. Such personal fulfillment will enable you to accept yourself and to deal more kindly with others.

DEVELOP A THIRST FOR REAL LIVING

Jesus said, "I am come that they might have life, and that they might have it more abundantly" (John 10:10). That means in fullest measure, and that's an exciting thought. It should make us want to get up on our tiptoes, as it were, and reach out for *all* that life has to offer.

The late General MacArthur reportedly carried with him through the South Pacific campaign a framed motto from which he often quoted. The author was Samuel Ullman. I have found it to be of great interest and help:

"Youth is not a time of life, it is a state of mind. It is not a matter of red cheeks, red lips and supple knees. It is a temper of the will; a quality of the imagination; a vigor of the emotions; it is a freshness of the deep springs of life. Youth means a temperamental predominance of courage over timidity, of the appetite for adventure over a life of ease. This often exists in a man of 50, more than in a boy of 20. Nobody grows old by merely living a number of years; people grow old by deserting their ideals.

"Years may wrinkle the skin, but to give up enthusiasm wrinkles the soul. Worry, doubt, self-distrust, fear and despair—these are the long years that bow the head and turn the growing spirit back to dust.

"Whether 70 or 16, there is in every being's heart a love of wonder; the sweet amazement at the stars and starlike things and thoughts; the undaunted challenge of events, the unfailing childlike appetite for what comes next, and the joy in the game of life.

"You are as young as your faith, as old as your doubt; as young as your self-confidence, as old as your fear; as young as your hope, as old as your despair.

"In the central place of your heart there is a wireless station. So long as it receives messages of beauty, hope, cheer, grandeur, courage, and power from the earth, from men and from the Infinite—so long are you young. When wires are all down and the central places of your heart are covered with snows of pessimism and the ice of cynicism, then are you grown old indeed."

PUT GOD IN CONTROL

Are you a joy-filled person? Joy should be a crowning characteristic of every woman—it's your birthright as a Christian.

Perhaps you are thinking, that's easy for you to say; you've experienced so many super-great things in your life that would bring you joy. But there's another side to the picture —when the glare of the lights fades away and all the publicity and attention come to an end, you still have yourself to face. Fame is indeed fleeting and not always the lasting answer to real joy.

I appreciate the words of a Christian friend who has known both public acclaim and public censure. She tells me that to her joy is more than circumstances; happiness is not dependent on what's happening at a given moment or what other people are saying or thinking. She finds true joy and happiness in having a right relationship with God so that regardless of what happens—good or bad—underneath is the certainty of his love and care.

All of us have known women who have this indefinable glow—who exude warmth, poise, enthusiasm and a kind of unrestricted joy in everything they do or say. And we can each have it. But we don't achieve it by demeaning ourselves to ourselves or to others (that's called false humility); it comes only when we put ourselves under the control of the Holy Spirit. Enthusiasm and zest for living are natural by-products of living the Spirit-controlled life.

Your Mental Processes

Someone has suggested an intriguing image for the action of our thoughts. He says it's like having a rubber ball on a string tied to the center of our minds. You throw it out, and forget about it, in the involved activities of your life. But each time you're alone, the ball bounces back, a reminder that whatever you focus your mind on most intensely is the thing that becomes most important to you.

Are there implications in that for the inner you? It appears that the things that really capture your imagination will ultimately dictate the direction your life will go. But we can deliberately program our minds so that the end result in our daily living is beauty of mind. Philippians 4:8 says: "Finally . . . whatsoever things are true, . . . honest, . . . just, whatsoever things are pure, . . . lovely,

. . . of good report; if there be any virtue, and if there be any praise, think on these things."

A great philosopher once said, "My mind is myself. To take care of myself is to take care of my mind." When we really understand the power in our mental processes, and the necessity, therefore, for keeping our mental attitudes under the Holy Spirit's control, then we are on the road to mastery of self.

During the last days of World War II, someone commented to President Truman that he appeared to bear up under the stress and strain better than any previous President. His answer was, "I have a foxhole in my mind." He went on to explain that just as a soldier retreated into his foxhole for protection, rest and recuperation, he periodically retired into his own mental foxhole, where he allowed nothing to bother him. I need just such a quiet place inside my mind, a sort of mental and emotional decompression chamber.

Medical science has proven that certain emotions cause illnesses. Who needs bitterness, hatred, resentment, envy, and fear in his life? Paul counsels that we are to be renewed in the spirit of our minds (Eph. 4:23). To do this we need to rid ourselves of lying, untruthfulness, anger, stealing, evil speaking, talking about others, bitterness, filthiness, evil thoughts (Eph. 4:25–31). The Bible talks a lot about our relationships with other people and what this can mean to them and us (see, for instance, Rom. 12:4–5; James 4:11; 5:9; Gal. 5:15). Peter warns that we should gird our minds for action (1 Pet. 1:13); and Paul expresses the concern that the devil would lead our minds astray (2 Cor. 11:3).

Jesus said: "Out of the abundance of the heart the mouth speaketh. A good man out of the good treasure of the heart bringeth forth good things: and an evil man out of the evil treasure bringeth forth evil things" (Matt. 12:34b,35).

The resources of heaven are ours to apply against the defects in character that we discover in ourselves. When we first start down the interstate of life we have such grand ideas about what's up ahead. Often, however, we are drawn onto sideroads that look awfully bright, glittery and attractive. We take wrong turns and end up getting deeply hurt along the way, and we lose valuable time. Many never get back to the interstate; others come to a dead end and just give up; some of us do make it back to the main highway and, with God's help, try to move on in the right direction. Life is a continual learning experience, and I believe God wants us to help others by sharing the lessons we've learned along the way. I haven't reached my destination, but I intend to "keep on keeping on." Someone once remarked to one of this country's well-known ministers, "Life is so difficult. How can a person live in times like this?" His reply: "Why not try God?"

ᴄ 7 ᴐ

Personality Development and Social Ease

Contrary to popular belief, not all Miss Americas are out-going by nature. I know I wasn't. Many of us have con-sciously had to develop the personalities that we now have and our ease in meeting and talking with people.

When I was a child of ten or eleven, I was very shy and tense about meeting people as I was extremely self-conscious because of my gangly appearance. Yet I was constantly being thrown into this situation. My father was a banker, and he often took the whole family to the many meetings he had to attend, not only in my home town of El Dorado, Arkansas, but in other places both in and out of the state. I learned at that young age how to talk to adults.

My self-consciousness stayed with me, however, on into junior high school. Two things helped me overcome the problem. I loved to sing, and my family encouraged me. Of course, I can still remember the awful fear that gripped me when I sang my first solo. I was a seventh grader, and the occasion was our junior high assembly program. The song was "A Dream Is a Wish Your Heart Makes" from *Cinderella* (perhaps an early prophecy of things to come). But in the ninth grade, two other young girls and I formed a trio called the Philidons (Phyllis, Linda, and Donna), and we sang our way through high school. We became quite popular on the local scene, appearing as often as three times a week at various civic clubs and community events. In this contact with all types and groups of people, we had to extend ourselves, and the opportunity to develop our poise was invaluable. I know no better way to overcome a tendency toward a fear of meeting people than having to get up on your feet and present yourself in either speaking or song. A tremendously expanding experience occurred for us when we won a county-wide talent show, the first prize being an all-expense paid trip to New York City and an audition for the Ted Mack Amateur Hour. An exciting trip for a fifteen-year-old, but a disappointing one, too, when they selected a bottle player over us!

No less important was the help I got as a result of being a very active church member. Every week in our Sunday evening Training Union, I was assigned a part on the program and had to present it each week. I also sang in church and school choirs from the primary department up.

Shyness before groups can best be overcome by taking advantage of every opportunity, no matter how small, to stand before a group and make an announcement, or, if you are an officer of a group, to preside at a meeting. As you gain confidence in your ability, you will soon forget about yourself and focus your attention on what you are saying and what is required of you to convey a message to your audience effectively. This same basic principle applies to becoming a successful conversationalist. Forget about yourself and concentrate on what is being said—the topic of conversation as well as the person with whom you are communicating. Of course it almost goes without saying, the best conversationalist is really the best listener.

SOCIAL EASE

Some individuals never enjoy mixing with people because they have never learned the basics about social ease. Here are important principles that I've learned to rely on in this area.

1. Relax—be yourself. You can't be something you're not 365 days a year! Work to develop a positive mental attitude

about yourself. Suggestions that will contribute to the total you are spelled out in the first six chapters in this book. Learning to apply them will give you confidence in your appearance.

2. Dress appropriately. Know the type of function you are attending and dress appropriately. It is always safer to dress a little more conservatively than to be overdressed. My motto is, "When in doubt, don't!" Today our standard of living is more relaxed and we are generally more casual in our approach. Wear something you are very comfortable in, and if you feel good about the way you look, then you can forget about yourself. Like that eye-catching book cover, good grooming attracts. Keep in mind: "Simplicity is the essence of elegance."

3. Develop a well-modulated, controlled, pleasant speaking voice. Your voice is a projection of your personality and an important factor in the immediate impression you make —on a job interview, in a selling situation, when making new friends, and in other vital relationships. One effective way to determine how you sound is to record yourself on tape or a small cassette. Listen carefully to your voice inflections, pitch, rate of speaking, and articulation, and determine your problem areas.

How you speak is just as important as what you have to say. I am not talking just about pronunciation and articulation, but also about tone. Nothing spoils the effect of an attractive woman more than a very high-pitched, nervous-sounding voice coming from her mouth.

What really constitutes the sound of an interesting voice? The voice of a well-adjusted, well-rounded person who is happy and vitally interested in life will be well modulated within his or her pitch range. For each person there is a particular placement on the musical scale that is best suited for that individual's voice—an optimum pitch. Variation in voice inflection is also important. Avoid a monotone; let the pitch of your voice rise and fall like the line of a musical melody as you give emphasis to what you are saying.

The same principles regarding your speaking voice apply when using the telephone whether this is in the line of duty, pleasure, or business. Remember, there is no visual element in telephone communication, so it is doubly important that your voice leave a good impression. Remember this the next time you call for a job interview.

4. Develop a good command of the English language. Slang expressions and foul language should have no place in your vocabulary.

As I traveled around the United States I found it fascinating to note and study regional dialects. I was amazed to discover that even within a state there may be regional dialects. For instance, the state of Texas has at least five or six different dialects—East Texas, West Texas, the Houston-Bayshore area, to name a few. At the same time, I quickly learned the need for good articulation and clear pronunciation of words in order to be understood.

One of my first interviews as Miss America was in St. Paul, Minnesota. Being from south Arkansas, I had a slight Southern accent, and almost the first question a reporter asked me was, "Do you plan to lose your Southern accent?" My reply was, "Well, not if I can help it." Most of us are proud of our heritage and where we are from, so I am not suggesting that you try to lose a dialect (unless you are going into broadcasting, film or the art fields); simply pay attention to your general overall effect and improve it if necessary.

5. Be considerate. Don't monopolize the conversation either in a group or with an individual. There is nothing more frustrating than to be caught with someone who never lets you get a word in edgewise.

6. Do your homework before going to a social event. If you are invited to a small party, check with your hostess to see who else is coming. This is not being nosy; it is simply one way to think over names and make associations that will enable you to be more friendly at the party. For example, if you know that one of the men at the party is an attorney, or that his wife is president of the local garden club, you will have a base from which to initiate a conversation.

You will no doubt be attending some functions at which you will meet strangers. Sometimes it will be necessary to introduce yourself and get a conversation going. Simply go over, making eye contact, smile and extend your hand. Some etiquette books say it is not necessary for a lady to shake hands with a man or woman unless she so desires, but I have always chosen to do that. The immediate human contact it establishes I have found to be very helpful.

7. Develop a good memory for names. When being introduced to someone, listen very closely to the person's name. Being able to call someone by name makes a tremendous impression and gives that person a sense of importance. You know how you feel when someone you really don't know too well, or may only have met once, meets you again someplace and greets you by name. The best way to fix someone's name in your mind is to repeat the name immediately upon being introduced. I also try at this point to make use of a word association to a name. For instance, if I have met a man named Woodman, I say to myself, "A man chopping wood." After you have concluded a conversation with someone, repeat the name again to fix it in your mind.

If you did not catch a person's name at the time of introduction, speak up immediately. Simply say, "I'm sorry, but I didn't catch your name correctly. Would you please spell it for me?" or something similar. Timing is important; after an hour of conversation it is almost impossible to say, "I'm sorry, I didn't get your name." I recall several such awkward situations as Miss America—usually at noisy airports where I was being introduced to a number of people at the same time.

There will be occasions when you bump into a person whose name you've forgotten, sometimes even at the same party. The very best thing to do is to simply admit that you've forgotten: "I'm sorry, I've momentarily forgotten your name." Or, often it puts people at ease when I say, "I'm Donna Axum—we met last week at the Nelsons' party and Jane introduced us." Other people forget names too, and this gesture is appreciated. Please, never walk up to someone and say, "Remember me?" This has happened to me hundreds of times, and it is very embarrassing. My response is usually, "Would you refresh my memory?" And if someone asks if I have met Diane Davis and I can't remember, I'll say, "How nice to see you," instead of a yes or no which may be wrong.

It is also wise to listen to clues your host or hostess drops in his or her introduction: "Donna, this is Jim and Betty Jones. Jim teaches at the college—you won't find a better science teacher—and Betty is a dental assistant." Pick up on that and you'll have no trouble conversing.

8. Never prejudge people. I speak from the experiences I have had as a former Miss America, but this holds true for everyone. Many times we have some preconceived ideas of what a certain person is like, particularly of persons thrust into prominence—the President of the United States, movie stars, TV or radio personalities. But this can also happen on the local level—the mayor, your child's school principal, a neighbor, your pastor. Stories we may have read about other individuals or comments others have made about them before we have had the opportunity to meet them can create an image that can distort the actual relationship. Others find themselves in a difficult position when they have to overcome these preconceived ideas about what they are "supposed to be" like. Give them an equal chance—you will probably be pleased.

9. Be an interesting conversationalist. Earlier I said that the best conversationalist is really the best listener. But it is also important to be a contributing partner in a conversation—to be warm, sensitive, and well informed. We are not only to be interested in others, but we are to be interesting ourselves.

How is this accomplished? The busy homemaker can become lax in keeping up with what's going on in the world. Motherhood is a full-time, demanding job. The busy working woman can shut herself off also. We need to be well read on current events, world-wide and local. When you find yourself bored with life and yourself, then it's time to take a cue and devise ways to put some excitement and enthusiasm back into your living. This can take many different forms depending to some extent upon your interests and talents. But you cannot possibly be an interesting person to be around unless you are taking an interest in what is going on around you. This means extending yourself beyond the garden and bridge clubs and things of that nature. To know only what is going on in the car pools and the PTA is to limit yourself. As good as the PTA and some of these other things may be, there is more going on in the world today that cries out for involvement and the positiveness of enlightened womanhood. In particular, the Christian woman's zest for living, hope for the future, and knowledge of today's society and how it all relates to the Bible is desperately needed. Give of yourself and you will be greatly blessed, but moreover, others will benefit.

The importance of not passing on rumors or repeating unkind things about individuals was demonstrated to me with a real wallop shortly after I was Miss America. I was in New York City during the blackout crisis in the mid-sixties and it was a most unusual experience to be sure. New Yorkers were never more friendly. At the moment the blackout happened I found myself in the hotel lobby so there was nothing to do but find a place to sit down. Everything was in total darkness, the candles not having been located at that point. Shortly thereafter a gentlemen sat down next to me and we began conversing. He soon detected my accent. "Well, what part of the South are y'all from?"

He was obviously teasing me about my Southern accent. So I went along with that and told him I was from El Dorado, Arkansas, the home of three All Americans and one Miss America. "Well, I've never heard of it," he replied. "It must be a little bitty town, but that is quite a record. Now who was that Miss America?

I answered back, "Donna Axum."

He quickly came back with, "Ah yeah, you know I didn't pick her. She wasn't the prettiest one at all; in fact, I like that Miss Hawaii. She was a real good-looking gal."

I agreed with him that she was very pretty. Then I threw in some very pertinent facts about the Miss America pageant that the average person wouldn't know—things about the history of the pageant and the fact that the judges interview each girl and that intelligence is just as important as inner and outer beauty. He didn't pick up on that at all and kept running me down (not knowing of course who I was). Then he said, "Well, it looks like we're going to be stuck here for quite awhile. We haven't introduced ourselves, by the way. My name is—" and he gave his name.

I didn't know whether to tell him who I was or not.

Finally, after a long silence, I said, "Sir, if I told you, I don't think you would believe me."

"No," he answered; "what is your name?"

When I told him Donna Axum, he yelled out, "Somebody get me a light, get me a light!"

I learned right then that if you can't say something good about someone and you are uncertain to whom you are talking, it's the better part of wisdom to refrain from critical comment.

10. Don't talk about yourself, your accomplishments or your possessions, unless, of course, you are asked. And then, be modest.

11. Don't name-drop, unless by so doing you are reinforcing or adding to a conversation in some way that will be beneficial for all concerned.

12. Work at developing the ability to put yourself in someone else's shoes. Try to see the world from the other fellow's angle. Remember also that little things mean a lot: a thank-you note when someone has been considerate of you; a thank-you verbally when thoughtfulness has been shown or expressed (don't take people and efforts at kindness for granted). Be gracious to friends and family, and remember that every person regardless of rank or position should be afforded human dignity. Make the world a happier place by your presence and influence, even in small seemingly insignificant ways.

13. Always look people straight in the eye when you are talking to them instead of letting your eyes wander around the room. It is more honest and direct and makes them feel as though they have your utmost attention.

Tips for the Hostess

One final thing needs to be said for the benefit of the individual who is hostess. Your home is an extension of you; it should therefore reflect you, your family and your individual tastes and interests. People will be quick to judge you and your way of life by the way your home looks and your graciousness as a hostess. A few simple things to remember:

1. Always greet your guests at the door. If it is necessary

for you to remain at the door, have someone nearby who can assist you in making introductions as other guests arrive. If your guests know each other, that problem is solved, but don't always assume that everyone knows each other or remembers names.

2. Move among your guests and make certain no one is being left out or ignored and that stimulating conversations are taking place.

3. Be well organized so that you don't have to disappear from your party for long intervals. Keep your plans simple enough so that this won't happen; or, if you have someone assisting you, go over the details of the dinner in advance. Make your preparations well in advance. Allow yourself sufficient time so that you don't appear at the party the last minute, worn out, with frazzled nerves. No party is worth that. Lightness of spirit—not the grudging how-did-I-get-myself-into-this-mess attitude—is what's required (according to Arlene Francis, a magnetic hostess if ever one existed).

4. As you move around the room, concentrate on each individual if only for a few minutes. Make each guest feel as if he is the most important person in that room, and I guarantee you will be remembered and thought of in a very positive manner. This is a number one psychological point in any situation. Don't let your eyes roam about the room, but make eye contact and give your total attention to that person.

5. Before your party look over very carefully the physical arrangements in your room(s). Try to arrange chairs so that they invite an informal conversational atmosphere.

An hors d'oeuvres table is a lovely way to make it easy for your guests to socialize. They can thus move about at ease refilling their punch cups and sampling your interesting table tidbits.

In Conclusion

Throughout life we are constantly confronted with situations where it is necessary to meet new people, greet old friends, business acquaintances and associates. Some of their opinions will be formed before you ever open your mouth, based on visual appearances—your grooming and your posture. The initial first impression is often a lasting one. Give close attention to this so that you appear as a confident person, not arrogant, but secure and well-groomed. This will help you in all these other areas related to development of a gracious personality and genuine social ease.

The Bible says it so well: "Let brotherly love continue. Be not forgetful to entertain strangers: for thereby some have entertained angels unawares" (Heb. 13:2). The many references to showing love for others is a powerful recommendation for the never-ending demonstration of this all-important virtue. If we are motivated by this kind of unselfish loving, then we need not worry about how we are coming across to others.

8

Dealing with Success and Failure

Success and failure—these are two of life's most basic elements, human elements we must learn to deal with.

Let's look at both categories. I believe that being successful should not be limited to the traditionally accepted definitions of wealth, prominent social and business positions, or high educational degrees. Success should also be determined by the goals, abilities, and limitations of the individual.

To measure oneself by the accomplishments of your neighbors or "the Joneses" can often have an irreversibly devastating effect on your self-esteem and motivation. Rather, your successful attainment of goals should only be measured against your own capabilities and aspirations. For example, the job of being a good wife and mother for some women is just as important as an executive position might be for others. To use a popular phrase of today's youth, "it depends on where you're coming from."

Strangely enough, the public has a tendency to equate the continued success of former Miss Americas by their pursuit of a major TV or film career. This was the ambition of Lee Merriwether and Mary Ann Mobley, and they have done quite well. Phyllis George has been extremely successful pioneering in the area of sports commentary because of her ability, combined with her charming personality and beauty. Others, like Bess Myerson and Marilyn Van Derber, are making significant contributions in the fields of consumer awareness, public speaking, law, and education. Shirley Cothran is now married and working toward a doctorate in guidance counseling. Most of us return to our normal lifestyles and continue where we left off. I must hasten to add, however, that during that year we learn, mature, and experience the tremendous responsibility of representing the young women of America. As a result our lives are never the same.

THE GOOD AND BAD OF SUCCESS

Like most of you, I have attained some degree of success in my life. Publicly and professionally the most significant accomplishments include winning the titles of Miss Arkansas and Miss America in 1964, earning my bachelor's and master's degrees from the University of Arkansas, and pursuing a successful career as a TV sales account executive and producer and co-hostess of a popular show called "Noon" on KTBC-TV in Austin. I attribute these successes to determination, timing, hard work, help from many people, and the grace of God. On this long road I've tried hard never to lose sight of my objectives.

As I related in earlier chapters, the climb to the Miss America crown was not an overnight success story. Indeed, it took five years of work to achieve. The first important lesson I learned in the fifteen prior contests I entered was how to be a good winner and a good loser. (I lost six.) In every competition of life always keep these two things in mind: (1) You have not achieved success entirely on your own—there have been many people who have helped you along the way. Acknowledge and thank them for their contributions. (2) Unfortunately, in most competitions there can be only one winner. Remember those who have lost, because it is never easy to lose. A gracious acceptance of congratulations and sincere consideration of your fellow competitors is a must. You will find also that, once you have become a winner, you will have to deal with that "green-eyed monster" called jealousy. My best advice is to simply know that this is something that inevitably goes along with being successful; accept it and deal with it by continuing just to be yourself. Eventually it is usually overcome. You are what you are, accept it and be proud. Remember, jealousy displayed toward others will only weaken you in the eyes of others and eventually destroy you from within. Unfortunately, there are times when success causes you to lose friends and often being beautiful can be very lonely. Being Miss America can be an asset or a liability.

A word of caution to the winner: don't get carried away with your own importance and constantly boast of your achievements. Other people quickly tire of this and you will soon find yourself sitting at home alone reading your scrapbooks and polishing your trophies. Lenora Slaughter, former executive director of the Miss America Pageant, used to remind us that we were in trouble when we started believing all the flattering comments in the newspaper articles. After 365 days of that your head could get a little swelled! "The crown should be as loose at the end of the year as it was the night you received it," Mrs. Slaughter counseled.

When you lose, be gracious no matter how great the disappointment. Congratulate the winner, giving your support and encouragement if possible. Then after the shock of the loss is over, take a constructive look at your strengths and your weaknesses and learn from them. For, you see, you may have lost the title or the race, but you have grown immeasurably from the experience.

BE PREPARED FOR CRITICISM

Every person who attains any kind of public acclaim, be it honor or public office, should be prepared for criticism. Expect it and be prepared for it; as the old saying goes, "If you can't stand the heat, stay out of the kitchen." What's most important, however, is to abide by your own convictions, and live your life accordingly. Once you attain a position of prominence, expect at times to be misquoted or have your words taken out of context, turned around and given an entirely different meaning by those whose primary aim is a sensational headline. Expect your personal life to be a topic of conversation. I am still amazed to read bylines concerning my life that are founded on hearsay, with no personal interview or contact of any sort. But it is against those few journalists who feel that their column has worth only when every word is written in venom, with destruction as its purpose, that I would like to register my strongest feelings. How unfair it is for a false image to be established in the minds of thousands of readers simply because of the attitude of the writer. It is uncalled for and hurts very deeply.

My purpose in mentioning all of this is to draw a realistic picture of what must be dealt with when achieving success. You will find both good and bad as the price you have to pay.

The Bad and Good of Failure

At some point in your life you will fail—and probably many times—for failure is a common human experience. Benjamin Franklin said, "Show me a man who has never failed and I'll show you a man who has done nothing." As we start our teen years we begin making important primary decisions concerning our education, college and professional pursuits. From our late teens on we are experiencing some degree of independence from our families and in some cases choosing a mate and establishing our own homes. All of these areas are critical; how do we know we are making the right choices?

Let me offer some guidelines. First, know the answers to the questions, "Who am I?" and "Where am I going?" It is very important for you to understand yourself—your talents, goals and limitations—before deciding on a profession. Likewise, it is important to know your likes and dislikes and emotional needs before deciding on a marriage partner. You must know who you are and what you want out of life to run the least risk of failure. I say least risk because of the unknown elements that may befall us over which we have no control.

The majority of my failures have come as a result of (1)

overestimating my abilities at the time or (2) not listening to my innermost feelings and not being true to myself. Let me explain further.

A few years ago I thought that it would be great to work toward my doctorate in speech. I enrolled at the University of Texas for the summer and began taking graduate courses as a special student. My status was to be changed to official graduate student after I had made the required score on the entrance exam. Here is where my ambition and determination got in the way of reality. I have a very weak math background and as a result could not begin to pass the math portion of the test. I took the test twice but failed to come up with the acceptable score. I made all A's in my course work that summer, but found that I had overestimated my abilities in the math area. From that failure I learned some of my strengths and also my limitations. In fact, one of my favorite sayings is that "the only real failures are those from which we learn nothing." If I had been able to pursue the doctorate I would probably not be into my first love, television, and I would probably not be writing this book.

A Blessing in Disguise

Although failure is sometimes hard to accept, it many times turns out to be a blessing in disguise. In her book *A Man Called Peter*, Catherine Marshall explains that "sometimes the Lord has to close one door in order to open another." Many times, when we look back we can see how some failures have proven to be a crucial part of a positive step forward in our lives. For example, upon receiving my master's degree in 1968, I inquired about a job at the University of Arkansas. Because there were no openings I was forced to look elsewhere for employment. I was very disappointed. I received an offer to teach at Texas Tech University and at the same time host my first TV show. This was the real beginning of my professional career and life today. An earlier example: I competed for Miss Arkansas twice before winning. If I had won the first time, I would never have been Miss America—I was not ready. Sometimes failure means that a better prize is waiting down the road.

But there was one period in my life when far more was demanded of me. Until now, the details of some of the events that took place then have been told only by the media. My reasons for going over the story again are twofold: it is the strongest illustration I can make that failures need not be the end of life and that you can withstand severe trauma when God is there. I hope also that others may better understand from our side the agony we had to endure.

THE SHARPSTOWN SCANDAL

I can still remember the quiet hush of the Abilene courtroom and how my heart almost stopped beating as Judge Neil Daniels read the verdict to the charge of conspiracy that my husband of two years, Gus F. Mutscher, was facing. "Guilty." I sat in stunned silence, desperately clutching a friend's hand. Gus, then Speaker of the Texas House of Representatives, had been indicted with two other political associates in what has been called one of the biggest political scandals in Texas history. They had been falsely accused of helping pass legislation that supposedly benefited Frank Sharp, a wealthy Houston banker and financier. Gus had bought National Bankers Life Insurance Company (one of Mr. Sharp's interests) stock with a loan from the Sharpstown State Bank (Mr. Sharp's bank). When the indictments came and word hit the press, the bank failed and we found ourselves $340,000 in debt to the FDIC and Gus facing a felony charge which carried a possible 10-year prison sentence.

I first learned of Sharpstown in January, 1971, on the evening of the Democratic Victory Dinner. Nixon was running for re-election and the timing for the announcements of the Federal Securities and Exchange Commission investigation didn't seem coincidental. There were rumblings that the governor and lieutenant-governor were also involved, thus casting a cloud of suspicion over all three Democratic officeholders. Upon returning home that evening, I remember asking Gus how he was involved in all of this. I learned that, without discussing it with me, he had borrowed these large sums of money to buy the stock—a community liability. I was six months pregnant with our son and I had just lost my father after a long battle with cancer.

The year that followed was difficult indeed. The press began a daily bombardment of stories. Gus was being harassed from all sides on a daily basis by the press, the public, and an opposing group who became known as "the Dirty Thirty" (thirty members of the Texas House who were generally considered the liberal element). As the press wrote a chapter each day in statewide papers, the chanting grew louder and louder—"Throw the rascals out!" During those times our faith was a major element in sustaining us.

We lived in the speaker's apartment within the Capitol building, just off the House floor. The close proximity meant living in that horrible political tornado twenty-four hours a day for over a year. It was interesting to see how some close "political friends" (legislators, lobby, and supporters) began jumping ship. They feared guilt by association and damage to their own careers. The lasting recollection is not of those who left, but of those who stayed. They were the truly wonderful people who stood by and openly gave us support, love, and encouragement. Their friendship and loyalty will never be forgotten by those of us involved. I would once again like to say a deeply felt "thank you."

In September of that year the swinging hatchet fell. Gus was the only state official indicted—someone had to be the fall guy. The trial had been moved from Austin because of fear of not getting a fair trial. It was virtually impossible, however, anywhere in the state of Texas to find potential jurors who had not heard about the matter over the past year. The Austin judge purposefully moved the trial to Abilene, a conservative town right in the heart of the Bible Belt. To make things worse, Judge Daniels was a self-taught lawyer who had passed the bar without attending law school. This placed him under additional pressure. The press, who had been building up to this for a year, were there in such force from all over the state that individual seats were assigned on the benches of the first two rows, names marking the spots. Jury selection took about ten days

and then the trial began. Back in Austin our children continued in their daily routines, sheltered from the turmoil
by relatives and friends. Our son, Gus Hurley, was a year
old and taking his first steps. Gus and I flew back and forth
every weekend.

Frank Sharp had been given federal immunity in return
for State prosecution testimony. Mr. Sharp's testimony was
to be that the loans from the bank had been bribes intended to assist in the passage of favorable banking legislation. Mr. Sharp testified in Abilene that he and Gus had
been friends, but he did not state that there was ever an
implication that the loans were considered a bribe. Based
on that and other circumstantial evidence, the jury found
them guilty of conspiracy after deliberating only two and
one-half hours. Ironically, the day the case went to the jury,
the press took a vote among themselves, and the majority
voted "not guilty." That same press broke the glass out of
the courtroom door as they ran to their courthouse press
room to rush their stories onto the wire.

Only after the jury had left the courtroom and it had
cleared of everyone but family, close friends and our attorneys did we break into tears. In a short press conference
one of our attorneys, Richard "Race Horse" Haynes, announced our intention for an appeal. Then we were escorted
out of the building to our cars. The crush of the hungry
crowd of press made walking very difficult as we left the
building. We had to use our own bodily force and that of
two bailiffs to assist us in making it through. Reporters were
sticking microphones into our faces and shouting questions
all at once. In fact, one Houston woman TV reporter hit
one of the bailiffs with her mike, cutting his head open. She
was taken to jail.

Sentencing took place the next day, and during the night
friends drove from Brenham and all parts of the state to
stand as character witnesses for the three men. The courtroom was filled to capacity with friends when Judge Daniels
delivered a penalty of a five-year probated sentence, jointly
agreed upon by the prosecution and Gus's attorneys. With
the trial over, we returned to Austin. Gus resigned as
Speaker of the House and we moved out of the Capitol. The

moving van had just pulled away and I was getting into the car holding my son when one of the more considerate of the Capitol press walked over with his camera and asked, "Do you mind if I take one more picture of you leaving?" All I could think of to say was, "No; please, you all have picked the bones clean—there's nothing left." With an understanding smile, he turned and walked away in silence. The nightmare was over—and we had suffered deeply.

We moved to Brenham, Texas, a small German community of about 9,000 which had been Gus's home and strong base of support. Against my advice and that of several close friends, Gus announced for re-election for his seat in the Texas House of Representatives. We all helped him campaign in his five-county district during April and May. Although Gus maintained fairly solid support, there were factions within the community working for his defeat. As the election date approached, tension filled the hot early summer air. Newspaper ads crying "throw the rascals out" bombarded the district, and we continued to receive harassing phone calls. Gus's yard signs were being stolen as fast as we could have them printed, and one evening we were awakened by a noise and found that barrels of garbage had been thrown on our front lawn.

The election resulted in final defeat by several thousand votes, although Gus had led going into a run-off. With that defeat died Gus's successful political career in state government. The most valuable asset that anyone in public life has is his reputation. Once that has been tarnished or destroyed, it is difficult to rebuild. The Sharpstown scandal became a page in Texas history books and the bottom had fallen out of our lives.

When "I Do" Is a Mistake

The months that followed the election were difficult indeed. The tremendous losses we had suffered left us physically exhausted and emotionally and financially drained. By July, I had developed health problems and had to undergo major surgery. One year later a second round was necessary as serious complications arose, followed by a series of x-ray treatments.

Three weeks after my first surgery, I reported to my new teaching job on the speech faculty at Blinn College in Brenham. During the one year I taught there, many friends extended great support and kindness for which I will always be grateful.

During that same year, however, basic personal differences between Gus and me, which had been masked by the fast and sophisticated political life in Austin, became very evident and began to weaken our marriage. Gus was a thirty-seven-year old bachelor when we met in September of 1968. Our dates that followed always took place in large social and political gatherings—seldom on a personal, one-to-one basis. We never really got to know one another as individuals. Our number one mistake.

I had been divorced for five years after a short-lived, unhappy marriage and felt that Gus would make a good husband and a fine father for my small daughter. The security of a home and family combined with a very demanding political schedule seemed like the perfect life for me.

My marriage to Gus meant making several basic personal sacrifices, all of which I thought I could make because of my deep desire for a home, family and security. One of the most difficult changes was giving up my lifelong membership in the Baptist church to become a member of Gus's Lutheran church. Although I went through instruction and confirmation, I had a very difficult time accepting the change—the churches were so different. My singing and music involvement came to an abrupt halt. It was like cutting off my right arm—music had been such an important part of my life.

For many years before our marriage, I had actively participated in numerous Miss America preliminary pageants as emcee and singer, but this was no longer allowed because it didn't fit the image of a politician's wife. Even an appearance on the "Tonight Show" with Johnny Carson had to be graciously declined. I was miserable when all of these elements which had been so much a part of my life were taken away. It is important that you know yourself well enough to judge how far you can go in making sacrifices or changes in your lifestyle that may be required in a marriage relationship.

Gus and I were also from different backgrounds—he rural/small town; I, larger city, with extensive travel, independence, and a more sophisticated lifestyle. As a result, I had a difficult time adjusting to life in the small German town of Brenham although the people were very nice. During the summer of 1973, I moved back to Austin and began working at the University of Texas. We were divorced two years later.

THE LIGHT AT THE END OF THE DARK TUNNEL

I feel that it is important to end, however, on a bright note. Gus served two years of his probation and was then released by the Judge for good behavior. He is back on his feet again, with a good, positive frame of mind and doing well in several business areas. He is also back in county politics, having been appointed to serve the remainder of the term left vacant by the sudden death of the county judge. When Gus ran for his first full term he was re-elected. I am happy for him as politics are so much a part of his life—he was lost without it.

By mutual agreement, Gus assumes the responsibility of managing conservator of our son, Gus Hurley, and I am possessory conservator. The two of them live with Gus's family in Brenham and are a close team. This was the most difficult decision of my life, but I felt that at that low time Gus needed the love and closeness of his son, who means so much to him. Gus Hurley comes to Austin to visit my daughter, Lisa, and me frequently, and Gus and I have a good relationship. It was the best arrangement for all involved.

I am now producing and co-hosting a live, thirty-minute interview/entertainment show on KTBC-TV, called "Noon." I also do television commercials, emceeing, and singing, and have also returned to the Baptist church. I am alive again and happy. And I thank God for bringing us to the beginning of a new tomorrow. The lessons learned from this long and tragic ordeal have armed us with a greater capacity for living through the darker side of life and a greater appreciation for its brighter side. Above all, I now know that failure is not final.

~ 9 ~

You Can Make It—Alone
(The Single Woman)

As little girls we played house and dolls and imagined what it would be like when we grew up. Most of us dreamed that we would fall in love, marry our Prince Charming and live happily and securely ever after.

For some, of course, this happens, but the reality of today's society shows otherwise for a great many of us. Statistics show that, on the average, a woman will spend about one-third of her life alone as a result of death, divorce, separation, or desertion. Many young women are choosing to finish their education and establish a career before considering marriage. My best advice to all, whatever your age or situation, is—be prepared to stand competently and independently on your own two feet when the time comes. (That's independent—not necessarily "liberated.") Here are a few important ways that you can prepare yourself for successfully making it—alone.

BUILD SELF-CONFIDENCE

When you find yourself on your own for the first time as a young single, widow, or divorcee, you may be gripped by the fear of uncertainty—uncertainty about your future and your ability to cope with life on a daily basis. This is especially true if you have not prepared yourself mentally, emotionally, and physically to assume total responsibility for yourself, and possibly children as well. It's important, therefore, to look at your particular situation and believe that you can establish a happy life as a single if you *think* you can. Develop a positive attitude about yourself from both outer and inner standpoints as discussed in previous chapters.

Acquire Education and Skills

In today's competitive job market it is imperative that you obtain as much education and experience as possible. As a college and university job counselor, I encouraged young college students to get experience in their chosen field as they progressed through school. On-the-job experience, combined with the classroom knowledge, places you in a much stronger position to get the best job. I would also encourage you, regardless of your field, to develop useful basic skills such as typing and bookkeeping. (This does not mean that you should end up in the secretarial pool.)

If you are a woman in your middle years with an uncompleted degree or no college credit hours at all, check with your nearest college or university for programs geared especially for you. The University of Texas in Austin, through its Division of Continuing Education, offers periodic seminars called "Women in Transition." They instruct women in how to make a successful transition back into an educational setting. And don't forget to check with the Career Choice and Guidance Information Center for help in "fine-tuning" your ideas about an occupational field and in learning résumé and interviewing skills.

If you do not have the opportunity for more education and have no job experience, then make a list of your skills and areas of volunteer service. Through various state and federal programs and agencies, you might find employment opportunities in areas of social work or those in which homemaking skills are needed, such as schools for the blind, deaf, or mentally retarded. Nothing is more important than knowing that you can provide for yourself. This is especially gratifying when you enjoy your work and can build toward a future.

In addition to your education, check into public courses offered by women's centers or other outlets on such subjects as handling your finances, credit, wills and estate planning, insurance, taxes, or basic car maintenance. With this kind of knowledge in your background, you'll be prepared and ready to handle most any situation. You'll not be faced with the fear and frustration of "Oh my, what do I do? My husband always paid the bills and handled all the finances."

MANAGE YOUR TIME

"A woman's work is never done"—how many thousands of times has that thought run through your mind as you've come home from an eight-hour work day only to be faced with cooking dinner, washing dishes, and taking care of a stack of dirty laundry! In addition, if there are children at home, you also squeeze in being a tutor, counselor, driver, mediator, and disciplinarian! Without a strong back, constitution, and skill in time management, you will quickly crumble under the physical, mental, and emotional load.

Again—set your priorities: work from a schedule and assign duties and chores to other family members. When you work as a team with everyone doing his share, you all profit. This also enables you to spend quality time together. In addition, plan ahead to fit special entertainment and events into your schedule and budget. And while you're charting your schedule, be sure and leave a little special time for yourself—it's essential refreshment.

CONTROL YOUR EMOTIONS

Because we are women, our daily lives are greatly influenced by the delicate balance of our body harmones. In addition, our sensitivity levels and emotional needs will sometimes cause us to make unwise decisions based on emotion rather than logical judgment. This is especially true just after suffering a loss through death or the trauma of a divorce. In both situations several stages normally occur: (1) loss and grief—of a mate or self-esteem, (2) anger and frustration with the situation, and (3) acceptance. If you can just hold onto your rational senses until you've made it past acceptance, then you are usually "out of the woods." During the first two stages you are extremely vulnerable emotionally. Be very careful at this point. Don't make important personal decisions such as remarriage when your emotional needs are dominant. Let the muddy water clear *first;* then proceed, using your best judgment. Rushing into another marriage for security or better self-esteem can often end in unhappiness and even greater problems. Take your time!

SEEK NEW FRIENDSHIPS AND INTEREST

As a single woman, divorced, or widowed, you will probably find that you no longer fit into your married circle of friends. In the case of divorce, your old married friends may take sides and make things awkward, or you may find yourself simply not included in a couples' society. Also, you are now considered a threat by many insecure married women.

Becoming a widow is far more acceptable in our society because your loss is a natural one, but you will still be faced with the problem of not belonging in a couples' world. You will need to accept this reality and seek new friendships and interests.

I have found that the church is one of the finest places to meet new people with whom you can share common interests and develop meaningful friendships. Most churches now have single adult departments geared to meet the problems and needs of the single adult/parent. Look for people who are willing to put yesterday behind them and focus on tomorrow. "Today is the tomorrow you thought about yesterday"—make it count. Avoid negative people who constantly want to dwell on their problems and who never find a positive note in life. They will drag you down.

Develop new interests and hobbies. Force yourself to get

out and enjoy life instead of sitting at home feeling sorry for yourself. Join a club, do volunteer work, or take part in anything that will stimulate you mentally. It will help pull you up out of the depths of self-pity and low self-esteem.

CONQUER YOUR GUILT

One of the hardest elements a single working mother has to conquer is guilt—the guilt that she feels because she is forced to be away from her children a large part of each day. Because of the cost of living, however, we are rapidly becoming a nation of child day-care centers. U.S. Department of Labor statistics show that women make up nearly half our work force and that 50 per cent of those women have children 18 years old and younger. Although you would love to be home, ready with milk and cookies for them when they return from school, you must accept the fact that your responsibility to earn a living for all of you is of prime importance. Children readily adjust to this kind of situation when they understand that it requires a team effort. Devote thirty minutes to an hour of your time to each child as often as you can, giving them your utmost attention. This amount of quality time usually provides the needed balance and affords understanding between parent and child.

The guilt that divorce brings is indeed hard to deal with because you may feel that your decision was a selfish one, made to improve your own happiness. It has been said that in a divorce no one wins but the lawyer and the children lose the most. This may be true, but I feel that children lose even more when they are forced to live in an unpleasant environment where nothing is shared by the husband and wife except the roof over their heads. This can be a terribly negative force and children readily sense it.

If a mother is to be of utmost value to a child, she must feel happy about herself so that she can be a positive motivating force for that child. Living with one happy single parent in a happy environment, in my opinion, is far better than living with two unhappy ones in a home filled with bitterness and frustration.

Cash in on Your Nonproductive Time

How much nonproductive time do you have? By that I'm referring to time wasted away when you are not engaged in work or a meaningful activity. If you find that you have several hours a week on your hands, you might want to consider part-time work that you can do at home or at your own pace. After all—who couldn't use some extra money these days?

Watch for ads in local papers describing jobs of this nature, such as addressing envelopes, making phone calls, etc. There are also several fine companies in the United States which will afford you opportunities for building your own business by selling their products. The Amway Corporation is a fine example. In addition, some companies offer excellent fringe benefits which are invaluable to the single woman. A word of caution is in order before making any investment or signing any agreements: please check out the company with the Better Business Bureau and with Dun and Bradstreet. Check their financial report and success record.

Establish Your Credit

It is extremely important for every woman, whether married, divorced, widowed, or single, to establish her *own* line of credit and maintain a good credit rating. Establishing credit takes some time, so begin now regardless of your marital status.

In October 1975, something as important as the vote came to American women—legal credit equality. The Equal Credit Opportunity Act, effective October 28, 1975, provides access to credit regardless of sex or marital status, or, later amended, race, religion, age, etc. Under this federal law, you as a woman have a right to: (1) receive credit in your own name, (2) refuse to answer questions about childbearing, (3) have your income considered on the same basis as a man's on a credit application, (4) have alimony and child support considered as income, (5) find out the reasons for credit denial. According to the U.S. Department of Labor Statistics and the Women's Bureau, some 40 percent of working women are single, divorced, or separated. We have already referred to the fact that a woman can expect to have a single status (unmarried, widowed, separated, divorced, victim of desertion) at least one-third of her life. Would you be ready to assume full financial responsibility should your status change unexpectedly?

Credit is extended to those people who exhibit an ability to pay and a willingness to pay. If you are married, you may wish to establish a banking account in your own name, using a household allowance and any other source of income as cash flow. This is important whether you are employed or not. Most department stores will now issue you your own credit card—some may, initially, place a dollar amount limitation on it which can usually be changed after a credit history is established. This is an easy step to take and will prepare the way for you to borrow money from a bank or any lending institution for such major purchases as a car or home. There may also come a time when you simply need to make a personal loan to cover your living expenses or education. It is important to be prepared for your every need, planned or unexpected.

If you are getting a divorce, do not expect to be able to obtain credit based simply on your husband's credit history. Many women have had great difficulty obtaining credit after a divorce, especially if they have not worked or are unemployed.

Single women starting out on their own should begin establishing credit also in the manner explained above. A word of caution to all—don't overextend your financial capabilities. It is so easy in our "plastic card" world to charge without thinking of your overall expenditures. A way to keep check on your charging is to file on a weekly basis your credit card receipts and keep a running tally of credit purchases so that next month's bills won't exceed next month's income. I also find it helpful to keep a weekly budget book, writing down all expenses. At the end of the month or year this is a very helpful tool in locating the areas in which I am overextending my budget. At the end of the month, you won't have to say, "Where did all my money go?"—you can see exactly where it went. This system will also be an aid in planning toward major purchases.

Another essential for every woman is a good savings plan. Put aside each month whatever money you can to prepare for emergencies, or add to the family vacation fund. It is also wise to build up funds for your children's college education well in advance of the time when they will be needed.

The federal law which went into effect June 1, 1977, now requires lenders to recognize women's participation in joint credit accounts. Husbands and wives who already have joint accounts can request that the account be changed to reflect both names and credit histories. This also means that when either one accrues a bad credit record, that record is reflected on both histories. If either spouse allows the account to become delinquent, that fact will become part of a bad credit record for both.

Once your credit is established, it is extremely important to maintain a good credit rating by paying your bills willingly and promptly. If for any reason bad credit information is recorded on your record or you are refused credit, under the Fair Credit Reporting Act you have a right to: (1) see your credit bureau file, (2) correct any errors, (3) write a statement telling your side of the story.

A creditor must now notify a consumer of action taken on an application for credit within 30 days. If the applicant is turned down, the applicant must be notified in writing of the specific reason for the denial or of her right to receive that information.

Remember, establish your own line of credit, pay your bills promptly and willingly and don't overextend your financial capability. The time may come when you will need access to credit immediately. Use it and don't abuse it. The law is now on our side; make it work for you.

10

Life Planning and Self-Renewal

While judging a recent Miss America preliminary, I asked each contestant to describe herself in one word. The girl who answered, "Indecisive," didn't get my vote.

Following the judging of that contest, another of the judges turned to me and said, "Donna, describe *yourself* in one word today." It took me only a moment to think that through, and I replied, "Alive!"

After feeling almost dead for a few years, I know that *alive* is the greatest word to apply to my life now. Of course it is impossible to predict our exact future, but I feel I have learned a few important things over the past thirteen years that have helped me survive and feel alive today.

1. Have a good relationship with God, the creator of your life and the universe.

2. Know that because you are a child of God your life has worth and value.

3. Seek to develop your skills and talents to their fullest for a fulfilling life.

4. Learn to know yourself and accept yourself as you grow and change with each passing year. You will change and these changes are normal.

5. Always be true to yourself when making decisions. Ask yourself, Is it right for me?

6. Have the courage to accept failure when it comes and to learn from it.

7. Remember, in the final analysis, you are in control of your life and only·you with God's direction can change its course.

LOOKING BACK

No other national honor puts a young woman on a higher pedestal than the Miss America crown. In retrospect I would have to admit that much of the time I felt like a monkey in a glass cage, with people constantly staring. Such curiosity is natural, but it still can be unnerving to be its object. One minute I was a 21-year-old college girl from a town of 25,000; the next minute I was a national personality whose every word made headlines. Good or bad, my life would never be the same.

How did I cope? First of all, I decided to just be myself as much as people would let me. You can't fake it for 365 days! Second, I had to accept the fact that I was going to be closely scrutinized and face the realization that I would have the responsibility for influencing girls all over the country. (I still feel the weight of that responsibility.)

There were times when I inwardly cried out, "Take me off the pedestal . . . I want to be down there with all of you." But you can never exactly go back.

Many people have asked me whether, if I could go back, I would enter again. My answer is always a resounding "yes!" My association with the fine people of the Miss America Pageant has been a source of great joy, love, and satisfaction for me over the years. I am in total support of its ideals and efforts to give young women everywhere a greater opportunity for growth and achievement through its annual $1 million scholarship program. Over and above that, it forces each girl to compete not only with others but with herself. Regardless of the outcome, the result is growth and self-knowledge—two extremely important elements in achieving a happy and successful life. To sum it up, participation in the Miss America Pageant system forces one to strive for excellence—the very spirit on which this country was built.

I am proud to continue to be actively associated with the pageant on all three levels: local, state, and national. For over half a century it has been the Cinderella dream of every little girl. Its popularity over the years I believe is founded in the classic American spirit of competition and the need for heroes and heroines. America needs the stability of traditions, and I am confident the Miss America Pageant is a tradition that will never die. It is one for which I am extremely grateful.

ETERNALLY OPTIMISTIC ATTITUDE

Winston Churchill often said, "I am an optimist. . . . It doesn't seem to be much use being anything else."

A positive attitude is like the spark plug in a car. You may have the most beautiful car in the world; you may have the key to it and know where you want to go, but without the sparkplug of a good positive attitude, you are not going anywhere.

Of course it's difficult to maintain an eternally optimistic attitude, but it is one of life's most essential tools. A negative attitude will not motivate you. Rather, negativism is so contagious that there is even danger in associating with people who are negative. That kind of attitude may rub off on you. Instead, think positively.

LIFE KEEPS HAPPENING EVERY DAY

Most people prefer to be around optimistic individuals. It is my nature to gravitate toward persons who have a positive viewpoint. A song that exemplifies this attitude is one Liza Minelli sings. It is called "Yes," and the lyrics go something like this: "Life keeps happening everyday. Say yes, yes I can, yes I will, Yes I am, and yes I'll be, oh, yes!"

With that kind of an attitude, you can tackle anything that seems insurmountable.

But how do you stay up all the time?

You don't, of course—and it is perfectly normal to suffer from occasional feelings of insecurity. I do; everyone at some time must deal with this problem. Feelings of rejection are also related and need to be dealt with before they begin to affect your life negatively.

1. Do whatever is necessary to improve your self-image and confidence.

2. Try to eliminate those people or elements that have a negative force on your life.

3. Seek out the objective counsel of a trustworthy friend who will serve as a sounding board and offer support.

4. Pray about it. These steps have helped me cope with my fears and insecurities through the years. Usually if you admit your fears and weaknesses, you can overcome them.

Out of the fragments left of my life following the events related in the previous chapter, I took stock once again of my situation. Deep down I knew that I did love life and all it had to offer. I knew that better things still lay around the corner. I decided I would not succumb to the downward drag but that I would go on living, restoring all those elements that were essential parts of my very being.

I have always loved and depended on the wisdom of some of the sages of the past. At this time of crisis, the words of Will Rogers were especially meaningful. He wrote: "We never lose so much that we have nothing left for which to give thanks." And then he said: "Don't let yesterday use up too much of today."

BE FEMININE, BUT COMPETENT!

I strongly feel we women should be prepared to stand on our own two feet regardless of age or marital and family status. As we talked about in chapter 9, to do this we can turn to our formal education, the development of skills we have pursued along the way, our own native talents and gifts, our hobbies, and all that we have acquired in the way of practical knowledge and experience.

Plan ahead. Learn to anticipate needs. Don't leave all the financial matters up to your husband. I really feel sorry for the helpless woman who is so totally dependent upon her husband she has never learned to pay a bill or balance a checkbook. Life could have some traumatic experiences in store.

Never rest on past laurels. What you accomplished last week or ten years or more ago will not carry you through the competitive world of today. Most women have a tendency to let their emotional needs influence too many of the decisions that should be made from a rational and more practical point of view. Develop good common sense—or "horse sense" as some call it—and learn how to make decisions. Carefully evaluate your decisions great and small. Apply these criteria in your decision-making:

1. Is it reflective of your moral standards?
2. Is it right for *me?* Be honest with yourself; you stand to hurt and lose the most in the long run if you have not been totally honest.
3. How will it affect my family and those I love?
4. Is it a logical step towards the realization of a goal, or a costly false detour?

"HELLO, HAPPY PEOPLE!"

There have been few people in my life that have inspired me more than a gentleman I met in 1965 in Lubbock, Texas. He called me one day and invited me to appear for his civic club. That was the beginning of a treasured friendship with a gentleman named Mr. R. B. McAllister. He and his wonderful family became my close friends.

Mr. McAllister was a fine Christian man, and he went about doing good things for many, many people regardless of their status in society. In addition to dealing with his own share of problems, he was constantly helping people who were less fortunate.

Every time he called me on the phone his first words were a cheery "hello, happy people," a phrase that he had used in broadcasting over the years. Regardless of how I might have been feeling, he always brightened my day.

Life was not handed to Mr. McAllister just the way he wanted it. At about the age of nineteen he contracted polio, and from that point on he wore a brace on his leg and walked with a limp. You noticed it when you first met him, but after that you didn't notice it at all. The thing you did always notice was his smile, and his positive attitude.

He was also one of the most creative people I have ever known. He spent a great deal of time thinking of ways to use my talents in radio and television and entertaining. He had been broadcasting for many years and gave me the opportunity of having my first television show in Lubbock, "A Date with Donna." So he meant a great deal to me professionally, but also as a trusted friend. I marveled at his attitude about tackling the impossible. He always said, "Don't be afraid to attempt something just because it seems insurmountable. Just take one step at a time, and many times you will be surprised that indeed it can be accomplished." And he did accomplish many monumental tasks in his lifetime.

As a member of the Texas House of Representatives, he made a significant contribution to public education legislation for the children of Texas. When he died of cancer shortly before Christmas of 1976, it was a great loss to all of us. We loved him very much, but we know that because of his wonderful faith in Jesus Christ that he is happy. I know he would be pleased to sanction this book. He made himself available to me for counsel and help, and gave much encouragement and advice when I needed it most. He was always there with that fantastic, positive attitude.

I think the finest advice he offered me came in a time of real personal crises. He encouraged me to pray about my decision; then make the choice, go forward, adjust to it, and live with that decision as a part of my life. Often as I have faced challenges and accomplished goals in my life, I have thought about him. I am so thankful for his friendship— he positively touched my life and the lives of so many others.

As you seek to order your own life, I would ask you this question: Can it be said of you, "Hello, happy person"? If not, why not? If not, what can you do right now to bring about a change?

Life Planning

Frequently we ask children, "What do you want to be when you grow up?" Traditionally the answers have been nurse, policeman, fireman, mother, and so on. Some children will follow through with their goals as adults, but others will change their minds many times. Here I would like to make two important points: (1) it is important to know your goal but even more important to know your purpose; (2) it is not abnormal to want to change goals or career objectives at different points in your life.

How often we hear people say, "If only I had done this," or, "If only I had tried that." Don't live in a world of "if onlys"; start making things happen in your life today through planning. Start now—right where you are, not with the triumphs and failures of yesterday.

In order to evaluate your life to date, jot down the answers to the exercises that follow. Give yourself time. Be honest with yourself as you take account of your assets and liabilities.

If you are not totally happy—start today bringing your life into focus by determining who you are and where you are today and where you would like to be in the future.

Exercises in Personal Evaluation and Goal-Setting

Exercise 1

Values are what you consider important *to you,* things you will take significant risks to attain. Since goals are values in action, it is important to know your value priorities in order to set goal priorities. Number the following values according to their importance to you. Assign *1* to the most important, *2* to the next, etc.

_____Affection—love, friendship, loyalty in personal relationships

_____Respect—individual recognition for one's capacity as a human being

_____Skill—development of physical and mental talents

_____Wealth—ability to fulfill material wants and needs

_____Power—involvement in making important decisions

_____Enlightenment—educational background needed to make important decisions

_____Well-being—mental and physical health

_____Rectitude—a sense of right and wrong (adherence to moral and ethical standards)

Exercise 2

This exercise is designed to help you examine your ambitions, your strong points, and your weaknesses. (There will be some overlap among sections.)

A.

List experiences that have given you the feeling that life is enjoyable and worthwhile—those that made you glad to be alive.

B.

List things you do well, even if they are things you do not like doing.

C.

List things you do poorly but which for some reason or another you need to do or want to do. Do not include things that you have no interest in or do not need to do.

D.

To help organize your thinking toward goal-setting and achievement, use the following four categories. Consider things you would like to stop doing, things you would like to learn to do well, experiences you would like to have. Include both long- and short-term goals.

Statement of goal	Preparations needed to reach goal	Realistic date for reaching goal	Problems to be solved

11

Priorities and Time Management

"I'm sorry, I just don't have time." Does that sound familiar? Chances are you have said those words many times in your life, especially if you have a difficult time setting priorities and organizing your activities. The important fact remains, however, that you can always find time to do what you want to do.

If you think that you don't have any excess time, why not take one day and jot down every two or three hours exactly how you spent that time. You are probably in for a shock. Most of us will find several wasted hours that could be used productively.

It's hard for me to remember when I wasn't involved in many concurrent activities—my work, church, choir, family, housework, civic affairs, entertaining, emceeing. I have learned three important steps over the years that make my life workable and still afford me time for myself, family and friends: (1) set your priorities, that is, decide the areas to which you want to devote the most time—family, business, church, etc.; (2) learn to organize your time effectively; (3) learn how to say "no!"

PRIORITIES

The following three steps are excellent for learning to manage your time: First, you must realize that there are only sixteen hours of useful time per day if you sleep an eight-hour night. To use that time productively, write down a list of your top priorities and number them in order of importance. If you have more than five, you'll never make it—cut it back to three or four. Now think about your long-range goals in each area and try to determine how much time should be allowed in each area to achieve those goals. Force yourself to look ahead, not just to next week or next month, but next year, five, ten years ahead. A charted course will carry you further than simply drifting through life from day to day.

According to your priorities and goals, learn to plan your days and weeks effectively. You will be amazed at how smoothly your days will go and how much you can accomplish. Before you begin, be sure to assess your limitations, both physical and emotional. Don't try to do too much —you will spread yourself thin and be effective in nothing. Know your own pace and plan accordingly.

PLAN AHEAD

Here are the two ways that I have found effective in organizing my time.

I work with a yearly calendar book, which gives me an easy way to plan in advance. I prefer the kind that breaks the day down into thirty-minute segments. First, go through and write in important dates to remember annually—family birthdays, planned vacations, school holidays, special business trips, and so on. Next, concentrate on weekly plans one month at a time. Fill in special activities that are scheduled and any special reminders to yourself. Then fill in your weekly activities that occur on a regular basis. Now you are ready to fill in your days' activities as they come. This takes only a few minutes to do and in the end affords you greater freedom because you have allowed yourself time to plan ahead.

Now let's get down to daily planning. It's a good practice to plan each day the night before or the first thing over breakfast in the morning. This gives you a point of focus. Otherwise you'll discover that all you've done by 11:00 A.M. is watch two TV soap operas and you're not even out of your nightgown yet! (This applies only to those nonworking women!) Jot down a list of the things you want to accomplish for the day and number them in order of importance. As you complete them, check them off—you'll enjoy the great sense of accomplishment! For those of you who are forever putting things off, I suggest forcing yourself to start with the worst task first; the others will seem easier.

I'm sure you're sitting there saying, "This is all fine and good, Donna, but what happens when unexpected problems arise—a broken arm, a flat tire, clogged sink?" My best advice—"Stay loose and roll with the punches." And never, but never, lose your sense of humor! As Peg O'Neil, one of my Miss America traveling companions, used to say, "This *too* shall pass away."

Learn how to say no. This is very difficult for some people, but essential; otherwise you lose control of your own goals and "the tail wags the dog." It seems that the more capable you are, the more you are sought after by others for endless PTA committees, fund drives, parties, etc. You must learn to keep your activity load in balance. To do otherwise is a disservice to yourself and everyone involved. It is very easy to overtax yourself physically and mentally. Remember the importance of a good diet, rest, and personal attention; all these factors are essential in maintaining a busy schedule. And listen to your body. When it says, "Stop—I'm at my limits," act accordingly.

Use your scheduling to organize your day, then move at your own pace. Don't let it be your master, a structure not to be broken, but do let it help you keep your days in focus and your long-range goals in perspective.

Remember—today will never come again. Don't waste it.

A Closing Word

The purpose of this book has been to share the experiences of my life with women of all ages in the hope that it can be the beginning of a more beautiful outer you and a more ful-filled inner you. It is my hope also that it will serve to moti-vate you toward greater self-esteem and accomplishments, therefore enabling you to realize a life filled with great happiness, peace, and joy. I feel strongly that God is using my life for that purpose.

"... May God keep you in the palm of his hand."